T0361694

GREED TO DO GOOD

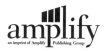

www.amplifypublishinggroup.com

Greed to Do Good: The Untold Story of CDC's Disastrous War on Opioids, A CDC Physician's Personal Account

©2024 Charles LeBaron. All Rights Reserved. No part of this publication may be reproduced, stored in a retrieval system or transmitted in any form by any means electronic, mechanical, or photocopying, recording or otherwise without the permission of the author.

The views and opinions expressed in this book are solely those of the author. These views and opinions do not represent those of the publisher or staff. The publisher assumes no responsibility for errors, sources, inaccuracies, omissions, or any other inconsistencies herein. All such instances are unintentional and the author's own.

For more information, please contact:
Amplify Publishing, an imprint of Amplify Publishing Group
620 Herndon Parkway, Suite 220
Herndon, VA 20170
info@amplifypublishing.com

Library of Congress Control Number: 2023923931

CPSIA Code: PRV0524A

ISBN-13: 979-8-89138-043-1

Printed in the United States

To Susie.

GREED
TO DO
GOOD

The Untold Story of CDC's Disastrous War on Opioids

A CDC Physician's Personal Account

CHARLES LeBARON, MD

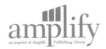

amplify
an imprint of Amplify Publishing Group

CONTENTS

FOREWORD

When the Centers for Disease Control and Prevention (CDC) announced that overdose deaths in 2020 had quadrupled in ten years, hitting a record high of more than 90,000, one opioid epidemic researcher exclaimed to the *New York Times*, "It's huge, it's historic, it's unheard of, unprecedented, and a real shame." He might have reserved a few of those adjectives since data from the following year indicated that the death total grew to well over 100,000, and the year after to almost 110,000. That's more than twice as many deaths as from breast cancer or prostate cancer or colon cancer, more than from automobiles and firearms combined. The cumulative overdose deaths this century now exceed the sum of all deaths for all the service members in all the wars of United States history. Within a few years, that cumulative overdose death toll is projected to double.

This book recounts in four parts the untold story of how the nationwide implementation of a seemingly simple, rational, plausible intervention by CDC had the paradoxical effect of turbo-charging the opioid epidemic. The first part is an in-person tour of the current narcotic landscape through my own painful experiences with opioids. The second draws on my 28 years of disease-control work at CDC to give a narrative insight into the unique institutional psychology that shaped the agency's approach to opioids as if they were infectious pathogens whose transmission needed to be interrupted. The third describes how CDC began its attempt in 2016 to control the opioid epidemic, applying that transmission-interruption strategy, and how six years of loud signals of devastating failure were ignored, during which period the opioid explosion became self-sustaining. In the fourth part, I describe the opioid control struggles of a Native American hospital where I was a physician, struggles both successful and unsuccessful, struggles that seem a microcosm of the national dilemma around opioids and its possible solutions. And in an Afterword, I bring these disparate stories into convergence to summarize what data and experience suggest about how we may be able to emerge from the cruel, lethal paradoxes of our self-inflicted opioid war. Which is really a war upon ourselves.

The language is the vernacular we frontline types actually talk to each other, and the book is part memoir, part history, part policy argument, part diatribe, part apology. It's an effort to tell a story where deep misery and high intellect and total foolishness, not to mention vaudeville and malice and even sweetness, coexist simultaneously. It's inevitably an emotional story about how we try, sometimes very greedily, very imperfectly, very messily, very politically, to use science to avert death and reduce human torment.

PART I

SEMI-PRIVATE EPIPHANIES

"Let us begin, then," she said, "with a few simple questions that will help in the diagnosis."

"Ask away," I told her. "I will answer."

"Is it your view that life is a series of chance events? Or do you think it has an order and a rationale?"

– Boethius (477-524), *The Consolation of Philosophy*

If everything's handed to you, you never get the chance to find out what you got.

– Mary Tyler Moore (1936-2017), actress

CHAPTER ONE

The North Korean Candidate

The afternoon of Sunday January 21, 2018, my girlfriend and I returned from a ten-mile walk, I made us some pasta primavera, we watched escapist television, headed for bed, read a little, turned out the light, and went to sleep. Around midnight I awoke with a fever and pains up and down my back. Tylenol didn't do a thing, I couldn't get back to sleep. Early in the morning, my girlfriend went out to get an anti-influenza medication, and that's the last I remember until I woke up in the intensive care unit three days later.

It wasn't influenza. It was staphylococcal meningitis, a relatively uncommon illness that has about a 50% death rate, particularly if treatment is delayed. *Staphylococcus aureus* is a virtually ubiquitous bacterium that lives on our skin and in our noses, where it more or less behaves itself, or at least does so while the body's routine defenses keep it at bay. If staph gets past those defenses into the interior of the body, say via a wound, it becomes belligerent, very belligerent. In my case, it somehow got into my blood and then into my spine and then into the lining of my brain, putting me into a delirium where I floundered about the house for three days in a high fever, falling on the floor, crying out in pain, knocking into things, refusing to eat, refusing to go to the hospital, loudly proclaiming that no one was going to take me to North Korea, growing weaker and more incoherent and ever more adamantly opposed to medical care.

Eventually my 27 year old son arrived, quietly told me that I was being impolite, keeping all those people in the emergency room waiting. Completely untrue – no one in the emergency room had any idea about me – but that appeal to good manners was shrewd. Even in delirium, even when life is extinguishing, we hate to be told we're committing a faux pas. With EMTs downstairs, I insisted on spending some time selecting a sufficiently attractive shirt color and style in which to make my apologies to the ER staff. Finally, I was cajoled into actually making that penitent ambulance trip to the ER where, having done my obeisance to the social graces, I indignantly regained my sense of personal autonomy. It took four people to hold me down for a CAT scan. Blurry with motion arti-fact, the scan nevertheless showed a variety of vertebral abscesses, one of which was impinging on the spinal cord in my neck and seemed about to cut off my respiration. I was far too rambunctious for a lumbar puncture without being put under general anesthesia, and time was of the essence, so blood cultures were drawn, I got emergently loaded with enough IV antibiotics to cover a whole textbook worth of pathogens, and I was shipped off to the ICU, restrained hand and foot and still raving away about North Korea.

In the morning, I proceeded to wake up, calm and a bit bemused, wondering what all the fuss was about. Where do you say I am exactly? And what day is it? Gee, all I'd really needed was that influenza pill, right? Isn't this a bit of overkill?

Amazing what a whiff of antibiotics can do. The blood culture drawn in the ER came back positive for staph, luckily the variety that isn't pan-resistant, I got switched to a single appropriate antibiotic, dispatched to a normal ward where I spent a couple weeks, then sent home with an intravenous line in place, suitable for getting months of antibiotic delivered straight to the right atrium of my heart. At the end of five months, other than having some fused vertebrae where the abscesses had been, making it hard to look up at the sky or do a full toe touch, it was a complete recovery. Whole thing apparently a mystifying random event, since my immune system was intact, and I hadn't had any wounds or other problems that would have allowed staph to get inside me. That mysterious random type of attack had been described previously in a bunch of published case reports. Reports in which the authors had confessed their mystification.

Fact is, we're all subject to the mystifying randomness of misfortune, whether it's staph meningitis or an out-of-control eighteen-wheeler or having one nucleotide out of 3.5 million nucleotides being "misspelled" so we have sickle cell disease. What are you going to do – apart from just accepting that randomness, just like you accept the randomness of good fortune? Even if the role of lethal, purposeless accident does gnaw on you a bit, the facts in this case were abundantly clear: this was a success story about excellent medical care and life-saving antibiotics. A very worthy kind of success story that does need to be trumpeted in an era when we actually debate whether or not some people deserve to have their lives saved because they lack resources or proper paperwork.

However, I want to tell a different story, perhaps less important than access to life-saving care, but one that may be less familiar. It's a story about the lessons that pain can teach. This is not the kind of pain that shows up in the one-to-ten scales devised by opioid manufacturers, or in the TV ads where joyful baby boomers play beach volleyball with teenagers after getting some injectable biologic costing hundreds of thousands of dollars or in the planetary massacres that we relish in action thrillers. No, the banal stuff, the pain we experience ourselves. The lessons of mystifying random purposeless pain.

Or, at least, what it taught me.

CHAPTER TWO

The Fugitive in the Abyss

Pain hurts. Pain's hard to define otherwise. You always end up in circular language, pasting different adjectives next to each other – disagreeable, uncomfortable, aversive, unpleasant, intolerable, miserable, etc., etc. Or we flee to metaphors of fire and knives and teeth – searing, lancinating, gnawing. Pain is just so irreducibly interior. We can tell someone else to look where we're looking, to hear the same sound, to sniff the same smell, taste the same taste, but we can't toss our pain over to somebody across the room and say, whatcha think? Simpler just to say pain hurts.

We need pain. People who don't feel pain in their limbs lose their limbs, and often their lives. But severe pain does hurt in a special way. It gets your attention. Unfortunately, science has yet to invent a pain-o-meter where people are informed exactly, unequivocally, and indisputably what level of pain they have: mild, moderate, or severe. (Look it up: those are the three official categories.) Then we could confidently have mercy on the deserving types and confront the malingerers with their fraud. However, even in the absence of a nifty little pain-o-meter, few in the field would disagree with the notion that acute bacterial meningitis and spinal abscesses might cause what could be categorized as severe pain. Sure seemed to me like I had severe pain.

If I wanted to sit up in bed I put a pillow over my face so I could scream uncontrollably. I couldn't even do a halfway decent job of writhing (the conventional physical solace of anyone in pain), since every motion of any part of my body made me scream some more. Even lying still hurt. I perfected the art of the silent shriek – where I yelled and yelled but the only sound was something a cat in heat might make.

This is different from the pain of running a marathon or climbing a mountain, pain that you choose. This is pain that's inflicted on you, that you can't escape, that pursues you tirelessly. You stare into an endless prospect that this split-second of agony will become minutes, hours, days, centuries, millennia, an infinity of anticipated intolerability, the inconceivable perdition that the fire-and-brim-stone preachers promised. Remarkably obliterative. Transformative. I couldn't read, I could barely watch television, I couldn't be distracted by soothing music, salacious gossip, slick jokes, sincere compliments, equally sincere insults, dulce de leche ice cream, fluffy service dogs' generous kisses. No attention deficit here. I was single-minded. There was only one thing in my mind, and that was pain. For those going through severe pain, the world is suddenly a mystifying place – how could this kind of awfulness exist in the world? And it's all inside my head? But it's the only place I have. Teach me the meaning. Or let me go. Please.

And then just to keep me on my toes, while my adaptive and innate immune systems were off fighting a life-and-death struggle with staph, a bunch of chickenpox viruses, more than half a century old, decided to take advantage of the situation by reactivating in my dorsal root ganglia and coursing down the sensory nerves from my spine to my skin, causing blisters all along the left side of my back from mid-chest to lower buttocks. And those blisters proceeded to ulcerate into wide and deep craters. This was a disseminated version of shingles, a condition said to cause pain as bad as childbirth. Never got around to doing childbirth myself, but I didn't find these widespread ulcerations quite as bad as that's supposed to be, perhaps because I was already a little maxed out on the pain thing. But all these ulcerations did make it almost impossible for me to figure out how to lie in bed without making things worse with my meningitis.

It was all pretty enlightening. *Staphylococcus aureus* reproducing in your leptomeninges or varicella zoster virus ulcerating your skin? They don't care about your pretty pleases with sugar on them, your heartfelt appeals, your promise to waddle on your knees to Lourdes and Fátima and Guadalupe and back again, your willingness to do anything, anything, anything! They're happily eating you. You're their food. They care no more about you than we care about the lobster for dinner that turns different colors while it struggles in boiling water.

In the movie *The Fugitive*, Harrison Ford (the wrongfully accused) stands at the edge of a giant dam, pursued by Tommy Lee Jones (the indomitable lawman). "I'm innocent," cries out Harrison to Tommy Lee, who replies gently, in a tone of great empathy, "I don't care." Whereupon Harrison flings himself off the dam in the hope of reaching a river thousands of feet below (of course survives and ultimately triumphs, an outcome not always seen in life). Stendhal said that the opposite of love isn't hate. It's indifference. And it's the supreme indifference that horrifies you in the pain – nobody can share it, you're reduced to total aloneness. Friedrich Nietzsche got it wrong when he cautioned against gazing into the abyss for fear that the abyss might gaze back into you. That's not the problem. The problem is that the abyss doesn't stare back. It's the terror that there's nothing in the abyss. It's the horror of facing impersonal vacancy, where it's all accident, it's all vacuum, it's all silence.

Yes, it's easy to get a little wacky, a little cosmic. Laugh if you want. But when you're there, you know you're in a universe of black holes and inconceivable distances and adventitious events, of which you're a meaningless, invisible fragment. The freezing indifference. Anya Krugovoy Silver, the poet who died of breast cancer in 2018 at the age of 49, had it right when she said:

> I have nothing to lose.
> If you push me off a building, I'll sing.
> I'd jump in front of a bullet if I could.
> I'd let someone wring my neck if only
> I knew it would hurt God just one bit to watch me die.

But it'd be wrong to give the impression that I had all sorts of sophisticated, rarified, metaphysical, poetical epiphanies there in that semi-private room I had all to myself in Pavilion 4B, with the perennial construction of a new wing making a hell of a racket outside, the fragrance of an unemptied bedpan, and somebody always insisting on taking your blood pressure at 3 AM just when you'd finally drifted into a dazed slumber.

Some must be ennobled by pain. They become truly exalted, radiant in their martyrdom, altruistic, self-sacrificing, beyond reproach, the person we all wish we could be. We have their examples throughout sentimental fiction, authorized biographies, three-hanky TV specials, 18th-century paintings of Roman senators, newspaper obituaries, lives of the saints, homilies from the pulpit, and addresses to cap-and-gown graduates, examples so frequent that they must have some basis in fact.

But I didn't find myself ennobled. I found that pain can diminish you in just about every way you can think of. I became querulous, demanding, self-centered, ungrateful, wheedling, cowardly, crafty, manipulative, sometimes all at the same time. Scant honor here, except for those willing to put up with me. It's amazing how you can shrink down to such smallness, your whole being reduced to I want, I want, I want. Kind of ignominious. You know it and you find that you can't do anything about it. You're reduced to animal mechanics. It's who you are now. So what's left to you? Narcs.

CHAPTER THREE

Puritanism and Pornography

Narcotics, opioids, those things do dull pain. They're also dangerous drugs: narcs can kill you, particularly when combined with sedatives. Plus (if that wasn't enough) there's a whole legal and illegal industry trying its best to get you to be a permanent, involuntary customer. True, there are a zillion other proprietary pain meds from which to choose, sitting there on the shelves of every drug store, and there's no lack of advertising to encourage you to take them – Tylenol®, Advil®, Aleve®, Voltaren®, Dolobid®, etc., etc. They work for mild to moderate pain (up to you to decide what that may be), they don't have an addictive potential, and it's harder (but not impossible) to OD on them compared to narcs. They have a couple problems: (1) each one is contradicted in the face of a variety of different conditions (as they were for me), and (2) they have a pain-control ceiling – past a certain point, increases in dosage produce no further reduction in pain but plenty of additional side effects, such as stomach ulcers, kidney failure, liver necrosis, strokes, and a variety of other things you'd prefer not to acquire.

So I got on narcs. For me, they didn't take away the pain, they provided an interval of respite, the world ceased momentarily to be scorched earth. And we do need respites to make sense of things, to understand. Yes, yes, all the great thinkers, all the renowned philosophers and prophets of past and present, all unanimously assert there are uses to adversity. Maybe. But I suspect those uses are almost always recognized after the fact, comprehensions only taking shape retrospectively when there's the luxury of just a little teensy bit of tranquility. Uninterrupted pain with no respite, no reprieve, sure seems uninterpretable while you're in the middle of it. Just like the hero of Dickens' *Hard Times,* who stares at the cold, distant stars from down at the bottom of a mine shaft where he lies fatally injured, the best you can say is, "It's all a muddle."

Well, I got a relatively high dose of narcs, 10 milligrams of oxycodone (popular prescription drug, popular street drug, popular OD drug) every four hours, a dose sufficient to deliver the pain-relieving equivalent of 90 milligrams of morphine. As it turns out, that's exactly the dosage said by the subject matter experts at the Centers for Disease Control and Prevention (CDC) to be the maximum anybody should receive. Maybe the max, but not a miracle. Definitely not a miracle. As it turns out, narcs create their own problems, particularly in the gut. At one point I didn't eat for four days, it was hard to get any Ensure down the hatch, my weight fell to the scrawny 140s (I'm 6'3"), and I doubled up periodically with really sharp abdominal cramps from the way oxycodone was slowing the peristaltic movement of my intestines.

But, more important, good old oxycodone did its primary job: I'd take the pill, wait half an hour till I experienced a fuzzy feeling that told me it'd kicked in, and then I'd make my move – first it was just getting out of bed (squealing into the noise suppressor of my pillow), a week later it was going almost to the bedroom doorway, another week and I could make it the six feet to the bathroom. Over the course of months, home by now, I progressed to the kitchen, to the staircase, to the front door. And, miracle of miracles, there beyond the frame of the front door was the outside world. That whole outside world was still there, so familiar but so new all over again, extending from the mailbox out to the bike rack and the street and on and on, all the way to the Belt of Orion and the Red Limit. There on my doorstep, hanging onto the jamb, I was silent on a peak in Darien.

Nevertheless, stumbling back to my bed, I got worried in my fuzzy state – high-dose narcs for months on end, what's the risk of addiction? So let's stop gazing in stupefied wonder at the Belt of Orion for a moment, review the lit, and put on our thinking caps. The risk of going on to addiction for someone given their first course of opioid treatment was said by a couple giant studies to be between 0.18% and 0.19%. Reassuringly precise, roughly a couple per thousand. But if you used an opioid for longer than 90 days, the addiction risk went up to as high as 6% according to another study. And then (according to still another study), for someone like me on high-dose opioids for five months, the risk of still using narcs a year later was 50%. Holy cow – 50% chance of being on narcs forever? No matter how we meta-analyze the scientific literature, we can agree, can't we, that I had thoroughly logical, evidence-based, and statistically robust grounds for concern?

You shouldn't agree. Let me confess: this is all anachronism. At the time, I didn't have a clue about these numbers. Who does systematic (or even biased, careless, and haphazard) searches of the scientific literature when you're waking the neighbors with screams because you turned your head the wrong direction? I was just plain scared of addiction. Not from studies, not from meta-analyses, not from my medical training, not from having seen the damage of addiction among my patients, but from glossy magazines at the supermarket checkout stand. You heard me right, the magazines in the rack right next to the tabloids revealing how a prominent politician adamantly denies having had sex with aliens. And fess up, you read the same stuff I do, while unloading your cans of soup. There's the star ending up in rehab after a Beverly Hills doc gave her a Vicodin script for a touch of migraine. And does she look like hell warmed-over now! Or how about the platinum-disk rockstar who got a pain pill for a dislocated guitar finger, promptly started shooting up heroin, then descended into bankruptcy, incarceration, and a final OD in a sewage-filled gutter?

But if it had only been supermarket magazines. Eminent medical journals were now publishing terrifying autobiographical admonitions, e.g., "My Story: How One Percocet Prescription Triggered My Addiction" by an anonymous nurse who described her dizzyingly rapid fall into addiction from a single opioid pill. Not to be outdone by anonymous nurses and supermarket magazines, the CDC Director was quoted in great, bold, double-sized font, boxed for maximum drama into an *Atlanta Journal Constitution* article: "If you take just a few doses, you can become addicted for life."

Hear enough of that and you began to conclude that opioids were not medications with uses, abuses, and dangers, but represented illicit pleasures, seductive delights that, once sampled, even the stout of heart could not resist. *Reefer Madness* redux – at the slightest momentary taste of an opioid, the unwary innocent who lacked superhuman willpower would be dragged inevitably to perdition. A single tablet dissolving on your tongue converted you into Faust signing his name in blood, demons cackling in obscene joy from below ground, flames flaring luridly across all the stage sets, a deafening, cacophonous surge of ominous music, and... doomed for eternity.

It's amazing how easy it is to spiral loose into panic when you're sick and in pain and in an all-round fuzzy state – your rational belief systems go wandering all over the place and get lost in frightening mazes of catastrophic thinking. You can spend your whole professional life scrupulously calculating numerical risk estimates for others and suddenly, when it's you (*me!*) none of that magic numerology matters – one Percocet, worse a few doses of oxycodone, and you'll end up panhandling under the bridge. And to tell the truth, even among the most autistic of us scientists, personal accounts always make a stronger impression than data. None of us ever broke out in tears over an odds ratio or a confidence interval. But give us shocking before-and-after photos of a fallen sitcom diva – blurry, ugly, paparazzi shots you flip through waiting to put your bag of spinach on the checkout conveyor belt – who could remain unmoved? *She turned into that? I could turn into that?* It'll haunt your dreams.

So there I was, with an abscess threatening to cut off the nerves that power my diaphragm, and what was I praying? Please don't make me an addict! Please! I don't want to end up panhandling under the bridge, please! Please don't make me into another Opioid Cautionary Tale! So many Opioid Cautionary Tales – please don't make me another! Then a few minutes later, the pain kicks into overdrive, and it's a slightly different prayer: forget the heck what I just said, we'll cross that addiction bridge when we come to it, I won't survive if I don't get my 8:00 AM dose of oxycodone a little early, maybe 7:30, I'll settle for 7:45, but the pain is getting worse and worse, I'll settle for anything, half a pill, you take the other half, doesn't matter, I must have some cash in my wallet, it's all yours. Go ahead make me into an Opioid Cautionary Tale – just give me my narc!

Now that's called being on the horns of a dilemma.

Eventually, I got lucky. Eventually, I wiggled off the horns of the dilemma. Eventually, the pain got manageable enough that I could wean myself off the narcs at home by slowly expanding the interval between doses, from every four hours to every five hours to every six hours, and so forth. Panting and grimacing and groaning, I'd call up people to help me do the countdown: only ten seconds to going exactly eight hours without an oxycodone – ten, nine, eight... zero. Eight hours without an oxy! Eight hours!! Then I'd grab the oxy and wait frantically for it to kick in and reduce the pain to where it was just a harsh part of my life rather than being the only thing in my life. There are better ways of cutting down on opioids in the face of ongoing pain. But sometimes silly behavior works just as well as mature, dignified, earnest, rational comportment. Maybe even better.

At the end, I was only taking a symbolic fraction of a pill a day. Now we're really into superstitious absurdity. Symbolic narcs. Ceremonially, I'd swallow a minuscule portion of a pill half an hour before taking a stroll outside. The narcs had escorted me through a long, long journey, saved my life in almost as many ways as the antibiotics had – so now somehow it seemed that if I stopped the narcs completely, the whole nightmare of pain would restart from the beginning.

One day, with great anxiety, I swallowed the last oxycodone simultaneously with the last capsule of antibiotic. Then I took a deep breath and walked exactly the same ten-mile route I'd taken right before I'd come down with staph meningitis. And amazingly I didn't wake up at midnight with fever and back pain, raving about North Korea. And I didn't feel some intolerable need to take another oxycodone. Nothing. I was done. Not completely done with pain. Who is ever completely done with pain? But I was done with the intractable, vandalizing pain, and I was done with that fuzzy stuff that I'd needed to make the pain manageable. Done.

Contrary to all the supermarket magazine stories and quotes from CDC Directors, I had been on large doses of narcs round the clock for months on end – and now I was off the stuff. No superhuman willpower against pornographic delights, no support group, no rehab, no opioid substitutions, no detox, it was all pretty simple. People who keep the tradition of fish on Fridays probably have a tougher time at dinner with cravings for that lamb chop in the refrigerator.

There are validated questionnaires – you put answers about yourself into a calculator (e.g., age, gender, alcohol use, sexual abuse, mental illness, smoking, legal problems, family history, etc.) and out pops your very own personal specific risk of transiting from use of prescription opioids to addiction. According to those questionnaires, my personal addiction risk had been pretty minimal. More anachronism. Who self-administers a scientifically validated questionnaire, derives the numerical risk, and announces they're wonderfully reassured – same time as they can't sit up in bed without having to shriek agony into a pillow?

How do you, gentle reader, think I got off the stuff so easy? Was it being the proud possessor of a low numerical addiction risk quotient? Was it my sterling character and steely resolve that made the slightest taint of unworthy comportment a moral impossibility? Or was it the fact that I hadn't felt any opioid euphoria whatsoever, just vaguely unpleasant fuzziness? Vaguely unpleasant fuzziness, abdominal cramps like a punch in the gut, total loss of appetite so the mere sight of food made me nauseated – quite a trifecta. When antibiotics had cleared the staph abscesses and the shingles ulcerations were healed, who in their right mind would want to go around with that opioid trifecta onboard? Or, maybe even more critical than having some sort of opioid metabolic processing variant that stopped me from lifting off to cloud nine, was it that I had good sociological luck? I wasn't unemployed in a town with rusting factories or shuttered coal mines. I wasn't navigating crime-ridden city streets where a dealer lurked in every abandoned house. Up and down the whole spectrum of clinical and public health, sociological luck is always the best kind of luck to have.

No matter which way you looked at it, I'd had lots of good luck: demographic, biologic, sociologic. And in every respect my luck had held. By the numbers, I'd had a 50% chance of dying, and I hadn't died. A 50% chance of ending up on narcs for years, and I was off the stuff. And far more important than avoiding death or addiction, I had dodged the fate of becoming an Opioid Cautionary Tale. Or at least the standard model of an Opioid Cautionary Tale, the kind recounted by supermarket tabloids and CDC Directors. But it seemed to me that I'd lived a different kind of Opioid Cautionary Tale – a tale that we rarely seem to tell each other, or admit even to ourselves.

CHAPTER FOUR

The Night Shift Nurse and the Subject Matter Experts

While holed up in the hospital, I somehow got on the bad side of a night shift nurse who decided to forget to give me my wee-hour oxycodone dose and wouldn't answer my increasingly frantic pushing of the call button. I wasn't a poor choice for that maneuver – I hurt too much to think about getting out of bed and charging down to the nurses station to raise hell. It hurt just to push the call button. Instead, at dawn, when she finally strolled in with the day nurse for end-of-shift sign-out, I was a simpering, whimpering, servile, sycophantic lump of excruciation – bygones be bygones, my lips are sealed, just please give me my 8 AM dose. It was a lesson. Who's in charge. And it ain't the person in pain.

But individual nurse orneriness wasn't my problem. I had made a bad mistake, really bad mistake: I had chosen to up and get myself sick in the middle of a nationwide campaign to reduce the rate at which opioids are prescribed. The year before, an Opioid Guideline had been issued by subject matter experts at my old employer, the Centers for Disease Control and Prevention (CDC), recommending that no more than 3 to 7 days of opioids be prescribed for acute pain. Only exemptions were for patients getting cancer treatment or those who were in end-of-life/hospice care. I wasn't exempt – meningitis wasn't exempt, disseminated shingles wasn't exempt, spinal abscesses weren't exempt. My acute narc dosing had gone on for longer than 7 days, even worse went on for longer than 90 days, and I was on narcs at a dosage that was at or above the CDC recommendations. Yeah, I didn't quite fit in. Turns out lots of people don't quite fit in.

If it had just been a run-of-the-mill CDC guideline, it'd have been OK. All sorts of CDC guidelines sit around getting ignored, particularly when there's no political will behind them, even when they're backed by good science. I'd written one or two of those myself, and they had sat around getting ignored. You could even say it's the fate of the majority of guidelines, no matter where they come from. We Americans are an individualistic bunch – we just don't like following guidelines. Even forgetting our oppositional individualism, those guideline things come out at a furious rate, two or three a week, from all sorts of distinguished or far-flung medical organizations, advisory panels, professional groups, governmental task forces. Always dense language, always tens, even hundreds, of pages with complicated tables, spaghetti-like algorithms, 12 billion references. Who could keep up with all of those things? As a primary care physician, you wish they'd just send a one-liner postcard and cut to the chase.

This CDC Opioid Guideline was different. Definitely not filed and ignored, not at all. It was even unparalleled in the speed and rigidity with which it was implemented, far and wide, by statute and regulation and policy, in both the private and the public sectors.

High and low, the people in charge were falling all over themselves in their haste to make it the Law of the Land. Politicians and media had suddenly discovered, a couple decades late, that there was an opioid epidemic going on. Now the authorities, the legal authorities, the corporate authorities, the network authorities, just about everybody but the illegal authorities, were going to make up for lost time by doing something about it. Right there on the nightly news. Virtue had saddled up at last.

It's hard to do much in a hospital bed while you're floating a bit on narcs. You try to watch a little TV, drift a little with any program, the shopping channel, two cheerful brothers updating old houses and selling them to happy, well-dressed couples, didn't matter, it was all Plato's cave. But it was amazing: no matter what channel I tried, the cooking channels, the jewelry channels, the dinosaur channels, I couldn't get away from authorities angry about opioids. Furious on prime time, irate at 11 PM, even livid during mid-afternoon news breaks from cartoons. They could barely control themselves on camera.

Lots of pictures of docs in mugshots, in handcuffs, in jail outfits, facing felony murder charges for prescribing narcotics. The U.S. Attorney General had just created a new "Prescription Opioid Strike Force," in order "to spot and prosecute more dealer doctors." The Georgia Attorney General's office had created its own version. The U.S. District Attorney for Georgia, surrounded by an impressive cadre of suits and uniforms, announced in a press conference that his office was sending out letters to 30 doctors who were "outliers" based on prosecutor monitoring of their opioid prescribing habits.

Accompanying that warning letter was a copy of the CDC Opioid Guideline. Easels showed the faces and profiles of disheveled doctors who had been rousted out of bed and arrested for violating the CDC Opioid Guideline.

Turn off the TV and have someone give me the paper, it was the same. CDC's hometown newspaper, the *Atlanta Journal Constitution (AJC),* was on a multi-article crusade, starting with the headline "Healers or dealers? Doctors and the opioid crisis" and driving home the point, "Well-meaning doctors who want to help patients in pain are part of the problem." Another *AJC* article in the series began, "About 1,100 of the state's physicians are now considered lawbreakers under a Georgia law intended to help put an end to the opioid epidemic, but so far nothing has been done to punish them."

"Punish" seemed to crop up just about anywhere there was mention of opioids. Or one equivalent phrase after another: "no scruples and no morals," "blatant sense of impunity," "feel they are above the law," "out of the shadows," "on notice," "full extent of the law," "stem the tide," "all the tools we have to bring them to justice." The Drug Enforcement Administration (DEA) announced it was offering free training entitled "How Doctors Can Avoid Being Arrested by Federal Agents." A DEA spokesperson tried to be reassuring: "We're not in it to take them to jail."

There, hospitalized and adrift in my narc and pain stupor, it was now terror between the bed rails. Beset on every side by these virtuous prime-time crusaders, how was I going to get my little oxycodone pill? The CDC opioid Subject Matter Experts, those CDC SMEs, my former colleagues, my peers, my old buddies in arms, they've all turned against me, they all seem to have turned into the night shift nurses. Worse than night shift nurses! The SMEs weren't just going to hold a dose. They were going to take away my oxycodone completely, leaving me shrieking silently into my pillow in a universe of pain.

Sensible, well-considered, realistic? No. Paranoid? Absolutely.

OK – but you give it a try. Try some ten-over-ten pain lighting up the whole inside of your cranium, and through a fog of desperation, you hear people talking righteously, pugnaciously, about how you deserved punishment and jail. You might get a little unhinged yourself. You might even think they're talking about you personally, the DA making eye contact with you right through that TV screen. You'd reach for the remote too. Just shut it off so he can't see me.

Fear of severe pain is a perfectly wonderful motivator, a phenomenon well-known to totalitarian regimes worldwide. Anticipatory dread is perhaps even more motivating if it's partially irrational, doesn't correspond to the cold, hard likelihoods. If you know exactly what's going to happen, you can deal with it. If all you hear are threats, then all you have is fear. And it's amazing the bad habits you can get into when you're terrified.

Before discharge, I spoke to my regular outpatient doc on the phone, mentioned my need for oxycodone, heard silence, mentioned it again, heard silence again. The chill, the deadly chill. Gotta switch docs, gotta switch, I thought. And did so. Once I got home, an oxycodone script went to my usual pharmacy. They wouldn't fill it because my girlfriend went to pick it up. I called them saying I was unable to get out of bed; they said sorry, I needed to show up in person for a narc. It was a rule, a good rule, a necessary rule. Oxycodone is Schedule II, dangerous, high potential for addiction and abuse. Hadn't I heard of the opioid crisis? Didn't you say you're a physician?

I found a pharmacy that would accept my girlfriend picking up the med. I called back to the first pharmacy. They wouldn't transfer the script: sir, that'd be enabling opioid abuse. They were shocked at my behavior. Shocked with an incorruptible tone. It's so nice to be incorruptible, straightening out the corruptible with all their smarmy wiles. Cato, Robespierre. I broke into hopeless tears, sobbing silently there in my bed, hardly able to move. Oh, how dearly I wanted to invent a little instant inter-personal pain-transfer gadget and say, "OK, here's ten seconds of the pain I'm feeling now. Not the hours, not the days I have had to endure it, just a convenient little sample of ten seconds. Whatcha think now, my friend?" [Various silent gleeful expletives deleted, some actually quite creative.] Unfortunately (or actually fortunately), that pain-transfer gadget hasn't yet been invented. So instead, I used my smarmy wiles and managed to obtain a completely new, duplicate script and get it filled at the different pharmacy. And luckily the state drug monitoring system somehow didn't detect duplication of a narc script, its explicit purpose. I'd snuck through the system. Outsmarted the authorities! It took a couple days to get that duplicate script. And in the meantime... if I didn't get that duplicate script? The Fear again. What if they catch up with me? I couldn't live with that pain.

I was already fantasizing ways to bring this whole messy, impossible agony business to an end. To a complete end. Complete. Tough to do when you're bed-bound, but there must be something in the medicine cabinet or cleaning closet that'll do the trick. What's under the sink? If not, what's the tallest building that has an open deck at the top? Maybe I could crawl my way down to an Uber, get to the building elevator, head for the roof, get out on the edge, look down 300 feet, think about how I was only five seconds to total relief, close my eyes, and...

Or maybe a gun store is simpler. I'll have to learn how to load the ammunition and take the safety off and aim at my medulla oblongata, that'd be the right place, or maybe the pons, midbrain. Don't want to just hit the cerebellum. Blasting out the brainstem is crucial. Got to do the job right. I'd feel around on my skull. Don't want to misfire and just blow off my nose or hypothalamus or optic tract or something and leave myself blind, pan-hypopit, and deformed. Good stuff for those continuing medical education credits required for maintenance of board certification, even if that certification has to be post-mortem. Yes, whole little unit on the extra-cranial landmarks for intra-cranial cerebral structures, should be sufficient for about maybe three of those credits. Two centimeters rostral from the mastoid process might be an ideal location. But vary a little too far sagittally... ? Dead is OK. Deformed and repulsive is really undesirable. But anything is better than trying to live another moment of torment.

Well, I did get my duplicate script and didn't end up going to a tall building or inspecting weapons in a gun store or trying to gulp down Drano. Soon as I got my sweaty hands on that little container of oxycodone, I gazed at the tiny white pills like they were diamonds, so precious, so irreplaceable. I couldn't let this happen again. So I began to skip a pill for one dosage cycle each day. Took some molar-grinding forbearance, some additional screaming into my pillow, but slowly I acquired a stash, a rainy day fund of these precious, irreplaceable little diamonds, hidden behind the vitamins, should the crusading DA and his SWAT team do one of those no-knock raids. Isn't that what financial advisers tell you is your top priority – always have an emergency fund? That was my emergency fund in a secret bottle. As time went on and my pain-control needs went slowly down, I made sure I got my full refill, despite not using it all – anything to build up my stash in case some CDC-inspired vigilantes attempted to cut off my pain meds, raid my medicine closet. Every so often, making my decrepit way to the bathroom, I'd peer behind the closet door – oh yes, there they were, so deftly hidden on the shelf, my tiny little round protectors against an outside world populated by night shift nurses and Subject Matter Experts.

It did get weirder. Picked up a couple pill bottles of oxycodone (by this time I was actually walking around), misplaced one somehow, angrily accused a pharmacy employee of having absconded with half my narcs. I'd read about that kind of thing in the paper, despicable people taking advantage of the helpless ill. We needed to review the surveillance camera footage, reverify background checks, do immediate urine testing, put the whole shift on administrative leave till we got to the bottom of it, and above all get me another container of the med that someone stole. Then I had to eat humble pie when I discovered the "missing" container right where I'd put it in the medicine cabinet.

What does this remind you of? Doctor shopping, pharmacy shopping, suicidal ideation, opioid hoarding, pain exaggeration, false denunciations to get duplicate narcs? Remind you of addict-like behaviors? What if rigid opioid prescription controls, prompted by the CDC Guideline, were provoking and even promoting addict-like behavior among those who had nothing but severe pain? Fact is, I had turned into a pseudoaddict. Yes, pseudoaddict, that's now an official term in the medical lit for pain patients reduced ignominiously to opioid-seeking behavior. Just like me. On the other hand, some scholars do deny the legitimacy of the term; they hold that people like me are actually covert addicts, cunningly and even disingenuously hiding behind the charade of pain. We're pseudo-pseudoaddicts. As we all know, nomenclature wars can get pretty vicious and personal, perhaps even more so when narcs are involved. Keeps people busy when nothing useful is being done.

But, whether I was an addict, pseudoaddict, or pseudo-pseudoaddict, I'm not sure that I would have behaved much differently if there had been a similarly draconian campaign against excessive antibiotic use, a campaign that might have threatened the thrice-daily infusions of cefazolin necessary to cure my vertebral infections. And fact is, from a public health standpoint, the justification for a draconian campaign on antibiotic overuse wasn't that different from that for opioid overuse. A study around the time of my hospitalization suggested that as many as 43% of all antibiotic prescriptions were potentially inappropriate. Antibiotic overuse had produced more than 3 million antibiotic-resistant-related infections and almost 50,000 deaths per year, more at the time than the number of opioid-involved deaths.

What if, lying in my hospital bed, watching TV, I'd seen docs who prescribed too much cephalexin being put in squad cars, pharmacies shuttered with crime scene tape because they filled too many scripts for doxycycline, states passing laws with strong penalties for anyone getting more than 7 days of amoxicillin? What if the same crusading DA, greedy for those prime-time voters, flanked by an impressively grim cadre of large men with large guns, announced on network TV that the combined forces of justice had broken up a Ring of Pediatricians who'd been giving out Zithromax® for runny noses? Whereupon the scene switched to those handcuffed pediatrician perps being led away in their nightclothes, trying futilely to conceal their faces? And all the while, there was a running commentary by well-coiffed anchors shocked to their very core at the depths to which so-called medical professionals could sink, inflicting the risk of unnecessary antibiotics on all those unsuspecting children who'd only had viral infections? What do you think? You're right, I would have done all the same ludicrous, dubious things to protect my antibiotics as I had done to protect my narcotics. For sure, I would have turned into an "antibiotic pseudoaddict." (Or "antibiotic pseudo-pseudoaddict," depending on which side you chose in a nomenclature war.)

But, off antibiotics, having taken my last symbolic quarter-tab of oxy, I was no longer an interested party in any nomenclature war. I was a proud member of the righteously abstinent upstanding world. I could look at the DA straight in the eye as he threatened hellfire and damnation through the TV. So I decided to get rid of my once precious emergency fund of narcs, proof that the pseudoaddict (or pseudo-pseudoaddict) phase of my life was behind me.

Turns out it's hard to get rid of narcs. To be clear, it's actually easy to get rid of narcs, you just stand on any street corner and wave a prescription bottle around and a generous soul in a muscle car with heavily tinted windows will eventually pull up and take it off your hands. Or more likely a homeless guy whom you can smell coming a block away. But I wanted to do this responsibly. There were stern warnings everywhere not to pollute the water supply by throwing narcotics into the toilet or endanger our children and trash collectors by throwing them in a garbage can. As a licensed, board certified, DEA-registered physician, I was going to dispose of these things properly.

So I took the container of remaining pills to the big pharmacy that had filled the prescription. They wouldn't accept them. Matter of policy: they didn't dispose of narcotics. They had been happy to profit by selling me the narcotics, but weren't happy to incur the cost of disposal. I went to another pharmacy. Same story, repeated over and over. As I learned later, this is strict DEA policy: once you get prescribed opioids, you're officially designated as the "ultimate user." If you don't want to take opioids anymore and try to hand them back to the provider or pharmacy, those folks are specifically instructed by DEA to hand the narcs right back to you and insist you keep them. If you're so obstinate that you leave without the opioids, it's considered "abandonment." The provider or pharmacy is then directed to "contact state, local, and tribal law enforcement or their local DEA office as soon as possible." Not clear what the penalty for "abandonment" might be. No guidance on what we "ultimate users" are supposed to do with those narcs we really, really don't want. But the message was clear: take those narcs or else.

At that time, little did I know that I was an "ultimate user" trying to "abandon" narcs, so I just googled up where I could turn the damn things in. Hmm... only a couple designated police stations. Not an enticing prospect. I still had some residual paranoia from those crusading DAs on TV. Scene flashes before my eyes: there I am walking into a police station announcing I had some narcs in my pocket. I'm escorted to an interview room where the chairs are bolted to the floor. Door shuts with a heavy click behind me. "Sit right down, sir, your driver's license if you please. We just need to check for outstanding warrants, parole violations, immigration holds, restraining orders, delinquent child support, unpaid property taxes, parking tickets, small claims court liens, unapproved zoning variances, septic-system overflows, truancy reports, excessive noise complaints, accusations of public nudity, overdue library books, the usual things."

Turns out, it was nothing like that. In fact, the cops were much nicer than the pharmacy staff, very pleased that someone was actually, amazingly, trying to get some narcs out of circulation. So welcoming was law enforcement that I wondered if I was the only person who had ever voluntarily made use of the service. *Voluntarily.* Why was I so surprised that the word *voluntary* was a word almost never used around opioids? Where had I been all my life?

CHAPTER FIVE

Breaking into Prison

We research-type physicians at CDC, or almost all of us, are required to do some sort of clinical work yearly to renew our patient-care skills. A good requirement, but not a popular requirement. It yanks us out of our cubicles where we're hunched over our computers, looking at numbers. Important numbers. We do those couple weeks' clinical work under duress, complaining all the way about this silliness of having to see unimportant sick people.

One year, having waited till the last possible reluctant minute to identify a place for my clinical time, I chose the local federal penitentiary. Purely for convenience – it was a nearby location with no credentialing rigmarole since I was already a federal doc. As it turned out, my clinical skills really didn't get renewed much in the prison, but years later recuperating in my hospital bed, with an indwelling intravenous line leading to the right side of my heart, worrying whether the night shift nurse would actually give me my midnight oxy, I realized a penitentiary hadn't been a half-bad choice for someone who long afterward was trying to understand the larger picture of the narc business.

This particular penitentiary was a formidable-looking edifice, built in the classic style of the early 1900s, with giant engaged Ionic columns holding up giant decorative arches of no discernable purpose and long, elegant exterior stairways leading to giant, permanently locked brass doors. Once upon a time, it had provided hospitality to Al Capone, Mickey Cohen, and Whitey Bulger, among other luminaries of crime. Rudolf Abel left it as part of a prisoner swap for Gary "U-2" Powers. Marcus Garvey resided there before being deported to Jamaica. Eugene Debs had run for president from one of its cells and received almost a million votes on the Socialist ticket.

When I arrived, those salad days were behind it, and this pen had the reputation of being the most violent in the federal system. A staff of 200 guarded 2,000 prisoners. Given shift work, days off, vacation, and sick leave, probably only 50 staff were present in the prison at any given moment. Prisoners did most of the work. You could stroll up and down the halls and never see a guard. Prisoner work was part of the mission, but rehabilitation wasn't. The primary, explicit mission was to segregate the prisoners away from the rest of society, through giant fortress-like walls and concertina wire.

Segregation might not be such a bad term. My visual estimate was that about 80% of the prisoners were Black. Since a Black male is commonly said to face a one-in-three lifetime risk of imprisonment, that probably shouldn't have seemed so strange. An equivalent proportion of the guards seemed to be Black, so it was really a relatively small number of low-paid Black men guarding a large number of unpaid Black men.

Several prisoner areas did have a higher proportions of Whites. The "minimum security" area (row upon row of bunk beds in giant halls) seemed to be populated mostly by Whites. And then at the other extreme, the "high security" area for the most violent offenders, where a guard had been murdered with a ball peen hammer shortly before I arrived, was also mostly White. And then way up in the "penthouse" (there was probably a more formal name for it), the high-profile prisoners were kept. They were all White. The penthouse folks didn't have to come down to the clinic where I worked. We made house calls. They were the hedge fund managers who'd run Ponzi schemes, disgraced public officials who were going to testify in corruption trials against household name politicians, organized crime figures waiting to go into witness protection, CIA operatives who had made a little money on the side selling arms to warlords. These were mostly urbane folks with urbane conversation skills. During a leisurely physical exam, they and I identified mutual interests, discussed cultural events and important artistic monuments of Western Civilization. Along with those urbane folks were a group of head-shaven, garishly tattooed members of the Aryan Brotherhood who had to be kept away, for their own protection, from the rest of the largely Black general prison population. To pass the hours, the Aryan Brothers and the hedge fund managers would play friendly games of cards. Or maybe it was whist.

Downstairs, the small prison law library (about the size of a CDC cubicle) had been burned down by prisoners protesting its inadequacy. The authorities decided to leave it that way as a lesson in the consequences of self-destructive behavior: Don't like inadequacy? Let's see how you like nothing. Perhaps an appropriate response, but the smell of smoke from the burnt library drifted everywhere, gave you the feeling of being in a war zone. But war zone wasn't exactly the right term. No firearms were permitted inside the prison.

Guards were armed primarily with notebooks, on the premise that the greatest deterrent to misbehavior was loss of prisoner time off for good behavior. In the cellblock that had been converted to serve as the clinic where I worked, the sole guard was at the end of a hall, about half a football field away, leaning back in a chair, chubby and bored and looking sleepy.

It didn't take long for me to figure out that prison medical care wasn't that different from outside medical care. You mostly treated the ailments of growing old. That's what happened when you were a prisoner: you arrived young with a mandatory minimum sentence for some drug-related offense, and you slowly grew old inside. You got hypertension, you got diabetes, you got arthritis. When you finally made parole, you had left your youth and health inside the walls.

But the world inside wasn't quite identical to the world outside. Everyone inside was on antidepressants. Everyone. Prisoners, guards, staff, everyone as far as I could see. Maybe even the guy who mowed the lawn outside the walls. No narcs were allowed for anything, but antidepressants were prescribed for everything. Everything.

Take lower back pain. There was a lot of lower back pain. Everybody did weightlifting. Everybody looked like an NFL lineman. It took a few days to get used to going into the crowded waiting room and find myself surrounded by folks who could break me in half faster than the faraway guard could wake up and flip to an empty page in his notebook. But the folks in the waiting room weren't there to break me in half. They wanted to see me. I was some weird doc who didn't belong there and had obviously wandered in by mistake. In fact, I was the only doc for most of the time, a fact that produced long, long lines for care. The regular doc was out for what was said to be uncontrolled high blood pressure. Or maybe sub-therapeutic antidepressant levels. I was in demand, if only for curiosity, check him out, he's that new doc, and he's only here for a while. I was entertaining. Novelty. It's mostly boring being a prisoner in jail. Very boring. Suffocatingly boring. And when it isn't boring, things can get considerably more exciting than you'd prefer.

One morning I was treating a soft-spoken young man in his twenties for acne. As was the case for seemingly everybody, he was there on some sort of drug charge. (Usual story of ambiguous innocence: "They said the stuff in my pocket weighed enough to make me a kingpin. I couldn't even spell kingpin."). He wasn't going to get out till he was nearly fifty, but he did have a girl who visited him and he wanted to look good for her. Maybe good enough so she'd wait for him. All his appeals were finished, but maybe something good would happen. Good things happen once in a while, don't they? What else are you going to think about if you're twenty-seven and won't see the outside of those walls till you're nearly fifty because you had some drugs in your pocket? Good things happen once in a while. Don't they, doc?

I was checking the formulary to see if they had benzoyl peroxide when there was a big commotion and a crowd of guards pulled me into the treatment room. Lying down on the exam table and shaking uncontrollably was a young man with a slit across his neck from ear to ear. The cut was very artfully done, the skin had been cleverly sliced, the subcutaneous tissue underneath was visible, but none of the critical structures below had been affected. Barely bleeding. So easy for that craftsman to have gone deeper, transect the trachea, sever the carotids, and the young man now on my exam table would have hit the cement then and there, foaming blood as he tried futilely to breathe, dead before anybody could do anything. No, this wasn't attempted murder, this was a delicately and adroitly crafted message. Apparently verbal admonitions had not been sufficient, so a little emphasis was needed.

I wasn't sure I could do that craftsman's work justice. It seemed like centuries since I'd done sutures. I looked over the materials. What's Vicryl again? What's Prolene? Which is non-absorbable? Is 3-0 finer than 6-0, or is it the reverse? How to do a forceps knot again? Could we wait till I can get some practice on an orange? The heck with it, I just got to work. Trouble was the young man kept shaking, wet with sweat and fear. And the guards kept asking him who did it, and he kept saying, I don't know! I don't know! Obviously he knew, but he'd gotten the artful message. Who saw it? I don't know! I don't know! Who has it in for you? I don't know! I don't know! All this yelling and shaking and interrogating and carrying on made it harder for me to do a good job approximating the edges of the wound, but on the other hand no one could blame my clumsy technique for what was sure to be a less-than-perfect cosmetic outcome. That scar was going to turn out to be a stark warning to others who disregarded verbal admonitions.

Eventually, the wound sutured up, they led him away somewhere else for more interrogation and I went back to my acne patient. I asked him if he knew anything about the situation. He didn't know a thing. The guards didn't know a thing. Turned out nobody knew a thing. This was the place where you whiled away your youth in suffocating boredom and messages were sent by sharp objects tracing delicate lines across your neck and nobody knew a thing.

I didn't last long. A few days later, there was a riot over the long waits for medical care, apparently a chronic concern. The authorities closed the clinic. Don't like waiting to get seen? Let's see how you like not getting seen at all. So I sat around in an empty office till my required clinical time was complete and I went back to my cubicle at CDC to hunch over my computer and look at important numbers, and didn't have to see those unimportant people who were locked up to keep the rest of us safe from drugs.

At this point, for those who may be as "opioid naive" in an information sense as I was, some stats might help. The United States has the highest number of persons incarcerated in the world. In the past 40 years, this number has increased 500%, in a period of declining crime rates but increasing severity of drug laws. In 1980, 41,000 were imprisoned for drug offenses; 40 years later, it was 10 times higher. And almost half of those in federal custody are serving time for drug-related offenses. Over the past 30 years, spending on prisons and jails has increased at triple the rate of spending on pre-K-12 public education. In 2017, the cost per year of keeping a person in state prison averaged $33,000, but ranged as high as $65,000 – or approximately the same as the yearly cost of sending the same person to Harvard. A lot of societal investment, a lot of taxpayer expense, a lot of imprisoned people, all to keep us safe from drugs. But who can argue with safe?

A couple years after my excursion into penitentiary life, the *Atlanta Journal Constitution* published blurry nighttime photos of people breaking into that prison. You read that right – breaking *into* prison. Cutting through the barbed wire and getting into the minimum security wing and thence who knows where, maybe even up into the penthouse. Breaking into prison. Every night. Laden with bottles of liquor and cell phones and goodies. Lots of goodies. The goodies you could swallow, the goodies you could snort, the goodies you could inject. Then heading back out before light of day with long shopping lists and detailed orders to various minions outside. A whole commerce going back and forth under the wire. Particularly important folks were escorted off to dine in nearby restaurants and spend the night in convenient motels with amenable local women, then courteously helped to wriggle through the fence before the morning head count. Most important, the business of goodies was alive and well, undisturbed by the fortress-like walls and concertina wire.

After that article was published, a strip search found 700 cell phones, or one for every two or three inmates. An enterprising fellow even used one of those smuggled cell phones to post a Facebook video, bragging about how he'd committed a murder. "Who done more shooting than me who's still alive?" he asked his viewers, laughing. Not an idle threat since this prison had more deaths than any other in the U.S. system.

A subsequent congressional investigation found, according to the *New York Times*, "widespread drug abuse, substandard medical and mental health care, out-of-control violence and horrific sanitary conditions.... Drug use is rampant, and unchallenged by staff members who either turn their backs or sell narcotics to the inmates themselves." The authorities were finally forced to empty out 90% of the inmates, after concluding that the prison had become a center for greedy international drug traffickers.

But in the larger scheme, it was apparent that the really greedy types, the major drug traffickers were nowhere near the Atlanta Federal Penitentiary, or any other penitentiary. They were sipping wine on Central Park South, sending their kids to New England boarding schools, bolstering our retirement accounts, and contributing lavishly to political action committees. Real scandals aren't hidden; they're just so obvious we no longer see them.

CHAPTER SIX

A Beginner's Guide
to Kick-Starting an Epidemic

Back while I was in the hospital with staph meningitis, the nurse's aide loyally asked me at every four hour vital sign check to tell her my Pain Score. My Pain Score on a scale of one to ten. I made a typical rookie mistake. I got factual. I said it was two when I was lying still, five when I turned over, went to eight when I tried to sit up, then hit an unbearable nine or ten when I tried to do anything more. "But what are you now?" I was always lying still for my blood pressure check so I replied, "Two." After a few days, the doctor got worried: "We're giving you high doses of oxycodone, but the medical record says you only have a pain level of two." I explained the situation. "Don't make it complicated for them," she said. Thereafter I got wise. I always said "eight" or "nine." Lots of people had gotten wise long before me. What narc seeker wouldn't say their pain was eleven on a scale of ten, even if they were laughing at a sitcom?

For decades, that Pain Score had been successfully marketed by opioid manufacturers as the "Fifth Vital Sign." And in 2001, the Joint

Commission (which accredits basically all health care organizations in the U.S.) had made mandatory a formal, documented assessment of pain levels for each patient at every interaction. So there'd be no confusion on what should be done about the pain, it disseminated a book for physicians' continuing medical education, in which it was stated "there is no evidence that addiction is a significant issue when persons are given opioids for pain control." It termed concerns about addiction "inaccurate and exaggerated." The book was sponsored by Purdue Pharma, the maker of OxyContin®. So in every exam room in every clinic, there facing you on the wall was a giant glitzy poster of a pain thermometer supplied gratis by an opioid manufacturer, with a happy smiling face at one end, red angry face at the other. Visible proof that you, the patient, were lucky enough to have medical staff who were caring. Caring about pain. Who's ever completely free of some sort of pain, small or large, somewhere, sometime, somehow? Who could be so inhumane as *not* to write a narc script to relieve that pain?

A decade later, the pain assessment requirement and the book were withdrawn with apologies by the Joint Commission. A little late. That was a decade during which there was a 100% increase in opioids distributed to pharmacies, a 70% increase in the average opioid prescription size, and a parallel 100% increase in the number of opioid overdose deaths. And during this same period, in response to manufacturer-provoked demand, the varieties of narcotics had proliferated into a cornucopia of opioid goodies – short-acting, intermediate-acting, long-acting, versions you swallow, versions you put in your nose, versions you put in your vein, versions that dissolve in your mouth, versions you put under your tongue, versions that you put in your cheek, versions you put up your rectum. When a cheap generic opioid was combined with a cheap over-the-counter pain reliever (e.g., aspirin, acetaminophen, ibuprofen) the narc doesn't sound like a narc anymore, it becomes a mellifluous bonbon like Percodan®, Vicodin®, Percocet®, or Combunox®, and the price jumps to 10 times as much as the two pills taken separately. From a profit angle, there's nothing like declaring that a proprietary version of a cheap generic opioid has an "abuse deterrent" feature. A month's supply of generic oxycodone costs $15, while the cost of Oxaydo® (oxycodone with an added ingredient to make it hard to snort) is $800. Both are equally addictive.

Aside from assisting the Joint Commission in promoting narcotic use, the Sackler family's privately held company, Purdue Pharma, entered the opioid hall of fame by promoting OxyContin® (a long-acting version of oxycodone costing 15 times more) as less addictive than the short-acting version, despite the fact that almost certainly the reverse is true. OxyContin® was given out in free 7 to 30 day introductory packets along with OxyContin® fishing hats and plush toys. Nothing like having your kids grow up cuddling advertisements for narcs on their dolls. Physicians with the highest rate of opioid prescribing were specifically targeted by Purdue for free trips to pain management "seminars" at delightful vacation destinations. In the five years following the drug's introduction in 1996, the company funded more than 20,000 such "educational" activities. By 2002, OxyContin® sales had increased tenfold and it was the most frequently prescribed brand-name opioid in the United States for moderate to severe pain. Three years later, it also earned the title of the most frequently abused prescription opioid.

But Purdue wasn't alone. The participants in opioid prescription promotion included much of big pharma – Johnson & Johnson, Allergan, Mallinckrodt, Endo, Teva. Take Mallinckrodt, for example: it had a market share of the opioid market 50% larger than Purdue and employed many of the same sales tactics as Purdue. Top executives from Insys Therapeutics were convicted of overtly giving bribes ("honoraria") to doctors to prescribe their product, a sublingual spray of fentanyl, the high-potency opioid most implicated in lethal overdoses.

All this was going profitably and transparently forward, right in the middle of the great "War on Drugs." So if you manufactured and hawked billions of opioid pills to clinics and pharmacies and doctors' offices, you made trillions of dollars and were a key part of everyone's S&P 500 index retirement fund. If you were an unemployed high school dropout selling a fifth of an ounce off a street corner, you got a mandatory minimum sentence of five years in prison.

Whether it was because of big pharma marketing, the Fifth Vital Sign, Joint Commission requirements, or other influences, the number of oxycodone and hydrocodone pills going to U.S. pharmacies increased by 50% from 2006 to 2012, capping off the era of what might be called the "Thoroughly Legal Opioid Epidemic." During that period, a total of 76 billion doses of hydrocodone and oxycodone were distributed, a cumulative amount more than sufficient to kill by overdose every man, woman, and child in this country. The linkage between opioid prescriptions and opioid overdose deaths began to become obvious: over the 14 years leading up to 2010, scripts and ODs had both shot up fourfold, in almost exact parallel.

And nearly inconceivable data started coming in from almost every direction. Pulitzer Prize-winning investigations by the West Virginia *Charleston Gazette-Mail* indicated that a single pharmacy in the town of Kermit (population 392) received 9 million hydrocodone pills over a 2-year period. Over 10 years, two pharmacies in the town of Williamson (population 2,900) received 21 million opioid painkillers. During the same decade, the state of West Virginia led the nation in its rate of deaths by drug overdose. In a nationwide survey, more than 30% of parents and 15% of their adolescent children reported that they had used prescription opioids in the previous 12 months. There was a doubling of the number of infants who suffered from opioid withdrawal at birth. Of persons recovering from surgery in the United States, 91% received opioids compared to only 5% in the rest of the world for the same operations. Even among postoperative patients reporting no pain whatsoever, 83% still received opioids. Of persons with prescription opioid overdoses who were lucky enough to survive the event, more than 90% continued to be prescribed opioids, with many suffering repeat overdoses.

It was hard to find somebody to take responsibility for this "Thoroughly Legal Opioid Epidemic." The pharmaceutical companies said they were merely manufacturing enough to meet orders from drug distributors. The drug distributors said they were merely distributing enough to meet orders from pharmacies. The pharmacies said they were merely filling prescriptions written by doctors. The doctors seemed to be remarkably silent. The buck always stops with the doc. Correctly so, since somebody needs to be responsible for the patient. But, is silence the same as responsibility?

Regardless, it was hard to deny that there was now an opioid epidemic. According to one study, the United States, with 5% of the world's population, now consumed 80% of the world's opioids. And over the first 15 years of this century, more than half a million persons had died of drug overdoses in the U.S., with the rate increasing so rapidly that within a few years the cumulative death toll might top 1 million.

Only one agency in the United States is charged with controlling epidemics: the Centers for Disease Control and Prevention. Where I used to work. At the time, it was the most trusted agency in the U.S. government. Epidemics: that's what CDC was founded to control, it's what it does all the time, everywhere, here and across the globe. Should CDC just sit around while this opioid epidemic, thoroughly legal or not, surges across America? Do nothing, just because opioids aren't technically infectious pathogens? Or should CDC get off its butt and go after the opioid epidemic? And crush it. Just like CDC had done with so many communicable diseases.

PART II

THE CAPACITY FOR FANATICISM

No one will ever thank you for a disease they didn't get.
– William H. Foege (1936-), CDC Director, 1977-1983

CHAPTER SEVEN

Purity of Purpose
and Unsparing Optimism

First, a digression, a necessary digression. Without an understanding of CDC's institutional psychology, so many of its actions around the opioid epidemic are going to seem inexplicable, even tragically farcical. This is a story of greediness. All of us can fall victim to greediness, and institutions are made up of people. But greediness in a public health agency is different from greediness in a pharmaceutical sales department or in a penitentiary or in a crusading DA's office. To understand the greediness with which CDC attacked the opioid epidemic, you have to understand CDC's history. Or at least the history it has constructed for itself. Each of us is hungry to be part of a story. Even better, an important story. Better yet, a history-making story. If you want to know what someone's going to do, listen to their stories of what they did.

The organization now known as the Centers for Disease Control and Prevention was founded immediately after World War II to execute a specific mission: eliminate malaria transmission. At that point, malaria was endemic only in 13 Southern states. The South, overall the poorest section of the country, certainly didn't lack for opportunities to make the same infrastructure improvements that had succeeded in eliminating malaria from the rest of the country. But infrastructure improvements are time-consuming and expensive. Was there a way to rid ourselves of malaria rapidly and cheaply? DDT had been called the "atom bomb of the insect world" by the military precursor of CDC – which proudly pictured a mushroom cloud on the front of a brochure proclaiming its accomplishment in ridding wartime Italy of malaria. By 1952, under the leadership of CDC, more than 4.5 million homes in the South had been sprayed, and millions of acres dusted from aircraft. Then came a backlash. Rachel Carson called DDT an "elixir of death" in her 1962 work *Silent Spring,* and 10 years later DDT was banned from the United States. But before that ban could take effect, CDC had managed to finish the job: malarial transmission had been eliminated in the South.

No governmental organization ever dissolved itself voluntarily, particularly one whose initial mission had been successfully accomplished. So new missions were undertaken – venereal diseases, tuberculosis, vaccine-preventable diseases – using the malaria elimination strategy as the template: launch a highly targeted initiative that focuses on interruption of a pathogen's primary chain of transmission at the most accessible point, and continue with relentless tenacity, even in the face of potential adverse effects or public resistance, till the goal is reached. Again and again, this strategy proved itself successful, with the domestic burden of multiple diseases massively reduced. So we got more ambitious. Why settle for one country?

In the early 1970s, more than a hundred CDCers were shipped to

Bangladesh to hunt down the few remaining smallpox cases left in the world. One CDCer described how such hunts were conducted:

> The initial stage in the evolution of a coherent containment policy was marked by an almost military style attack on infected villages... In the hit-and-run excitement of such a campaign, women and children were often pulled out from under beds, from behind doors, from within latrines, etc. People were chased and, when caught, vaccinated.... When they ran, we chased. When they locked their doors, we broke down their doors and vaccinated them.

Raids were made in the middle of the night; husbands grabbed axes to defend their families, but were disarmed and pinned to the ground, their wives and children forcibly vaccinated before their eyes; then the family was left to recover behind the broken door of their hut. A noisy enterprise, much commotion, loud commands in the dark, flashlights shining in people's eyes. Eventually, the whole village was vaccinated. Their choice: voluntarily or forcibly. Then the CDC team got in their cars and moved on to the next village to do the same thing. Wrote a different CDCer, "I was awful in my conviction of purity of purpose." On May 8, 1980, smallpox was certified as eradicated from the planet, and smallpox vaccination was stopped worldwide, the first such disease to be eradicated in human history.

No reason to stop with smallpox. A long list of pathogens was drawn up, each targeted for global eradication. The identity, the nature of the pathogen was irrelevant – the essential factor, the critical factor, was not the pathogen but – as one of the architects of the eradication movement had so succinctly put it – our own "capacity for fanaticism." The methods may have become more diplomatic, but that spirit hasn't been lost.

A hundred or so wild polio cases are thought to remain in the war zones of Afghanistan and Pakistan. In an effort to eradicate those hundred or so cases, CDC, in its fiscal year 2023 operating budget for global health, spent almost four times more than on all other vaccine-preventable diseases combined (>700,000 deaths globally per year), 40% more than on the global HIV program (1 million deaths per year), six times more than on malaria (1 million deaths per year). This is in a context of 1.7 million deaths globally from tuberculosis and half a million deaths from diarrheal diseases annually, with 9.5 million children under age five dying each year from preventable causes. The polio eradication operating budget exceeded the individual operating budgets for a long list of CDC's domestic programs, e.g., sexually transmitted infections (2.5 million cases yearly), foodborne illnesses (37 million cases), and cardiovascular disease (610,000 deaths).

We may be a quarter-century past the original goal of eradicating polio by the year 2000 – but we are down to the last 0.01% of cases. We're at the finish line. Trouble is, we've been down to the last 0.01% every year for the last couple decades. The last 0.01% is always tougher than the preceding 99.99%. It's estimated it'll take many more years and many more billions of dollars to eliminate those last few cases and cross the finish line. During which time millions of lives will have been lost that could have been saved if those same efforts and resources had been put into denting a couple of the big public health killers. Patience – the time of those killers will come. Once we get past polio, we'll go to the next individual pathogen on the list and do the same thing all over again from scratch. However many decades, or generations, or even longer, it takes. Pathogen by individual pathogen we'll rid the world of disease. Don't you want to be part of something greater than yourself?

To keep on task in a context where gratification is always just around the corner, where the pitfalls of demoralization and defeatism are ever present, you need the right mind-set. In public health, as in sports, it's all psychological. This is where the capacity for fanaticism comes in. All of us can become fanatics. We just have to find it within ourselves.

This isn't a matter of appearances. Institutions are only a bunch of people, and we bunch of disease control people sure don't look like fanatics. We look like we belong in H&R Block, all we lack are green eyeshades and pocket-protectors and well-sharpened #2 pencils all in a line on a desk blotter. There's a stereotype about us, rarely true in all respects but often true in some respects. We're overqualified for any position for which we might apply, toting about all sorts of semi-redundant degrees and certifications as if we'd been awfully reluctant to leave the dorm room and get a real job. You'd never pick one of us out in a crowd. We're not sharp dressers, makeup is as nonexistent as jewelry, don't bother searching for exotic tattoos. Weekdays, many of us wear the drab khaki uniform of the U.S. Public Health Service. Every Saturday night we wash that uniform, whether it needs it or not. Then hang it up to dry Sunday, so it'll be nice and wrinkle-free when we take it to work on a hanger Monday morning. Comparatively late in life, we find a sensible partner with a good work ethic, live in non-ostentatious homes in a neighborhood close to work. We save frugally, but it'd be very hard to corrupt us with money. Money's for a used Volvo and an index fund. But we have those already. So what would we do with money?

There are very few photos of us dancing on barroom tables.

Conversation at parties consists almost entirely of shoptalk. We only laugh at jokes when someone tells us it's a joke. We don't do irony, we ponder why someone would fall into the error of exaggeration. Explain something to us by analogy and we're mystified. We're not well read, so don't plague us with too many obscure cultural references. Music occasionally interests us if it sounds mathematical, maybe the Goldberg Variations. Drag us to a museum and we gravitate to the cubists, the minimalists. Mythological references elude us. Oil portraits seem like a quaint technology.

Send us to a city we've never visited, a foreign country we've never heard of, and we never study up on its politics, peoples, languages. Even if we stay for months or years. We arrive, we do our job, we come home. We weren't put down here to have remarkable realizations or tender feelings. We were put here to do something. We were put here to carry out a mission to improve the world, save it. Take away our mission to improve, save the world and anomie sets in, our universe becomes dull and meaningless, we sleep-walk through our daily lives with dazed eyes and miserable souls. We each need to add our own personal, illustrative footnote to the great history of public health. The story that tells us who we are. Not someone else's story – to feel it, to be part of it, to find your inner fanaticism, it has to be your own story.

So I arrive one morning at a decrepit building in Lower Manhattan. That's where the underfunded and understaffed NYC Bureau of Immunization is located, along with a bunch of other underfunded and understaffed bureaus. I try to go up the creaky, mis-angled stairs but get waved back by a man sitting at a desk in the dimness of the next landing. The landing is his office. He doesn't like people coming and going through his office. He motions me back down to a tiny, rickety elevator. I get on, right after a heavyset man. The heavyset man seems very unhappy. The elevator makes a lot of noise and gets stuck between floors. The heavy-set man says this happens all the time – when a second person is irresponsible enough to get on the elevator. Doleful expression. I try to look repentant. He pries apart the elevator doors. We can see the ankles of people walking about on the next floor. He looks at me expectantly. I get the hint. I lace my hands together. He puts a foot on my hands and crawls through the gap and disappears. No helping hand for me. It's hard being the culpable party. But the elevator had risen a few feet after he'd left. I'm able to wriggle up through the gap. As I do so, the elevator, released from any weight, tosses me in a semi-somersault onto the floor of the Bureau of Immunization. I'm lying amid what seems to be a zillion files, files of the thousands of measles cases yet to be investigated or reported. Everyone's going about their business, unperturbed by my manner of entrance, which must have been a frequent occurrence.

I dust myself off, stand up, and introduce myself to a person sitting at the nearest desk. "Hi, I'm from CDC," I say. She barely looks up. New Yorkers are hard to impress. Then with a sigh she pushes aside some charts. "We know," she says and shows me the giant tabloid front-page headline of the *Daily News* (at the time the newspaper with the largest circulation in the nation): "Ninth Measles Death! Fed Doc Arrives!!" From all sorts of sources, CDC knew there was an outbreak of thousands of measles cases in New York, but the Bureau of Immunization had reported two. Not two thousand. Two. Two cases, but nine deaths. Definitely a fuzzy mathematics problem. The city authorities had been understandably reluctant to invite anybody from CDC to decipher that fuzzy math. After some forceful encouragement, the invitation had finally come through, and there I was, dusting myself off amid thousands of files, trying to look just a little like the Fed Doc.

Alas, much to the disappointment of the millions of *Daily News* readers and those used to Hollywood action films, this particular Fed Doc wasn't able to help stamp out the epidemic by tomorrow's deadline. Or for a couple years. More than 85% of the measles cases were among Black or Hispanic children, nearly all lived in poverty, and nearly all were unvaccinated. At one point I was in a fruitless search for a map of measles incidence. I happened to be going through a state office building when I saw a perfectly beautiful map with all the high-intensity measles zones in hot red – the South Bronx, East Harlem, Bedford Stuyvesant. I asked a man in a nearby cubicle where he'd gotten that measles map. "That's not measles," he said. "That's the murder rate." Should have known. It could have been the infant mortality rate, the rodent infestation rate, the school dropout rate, the malnutrition rate, the incarceration rate, the premature-baby rate, the substandard-housing rate, the five-alarm-fire rate, or anything else in the misery category. Such as the opioid overdose rate. In public health, it's almost always the same map.

But at CDC, you're not there to solve the murder rate and the infant mortality rate and the rodent infestation rate and everything else. You're not there to solve everything. It's the measles epidemic. That's why you're there, dude, not the rodents. Repairing the infrastructure, getting rid of the rodents, takes time. In an epidemic, you don't take your time. Particularly when you have a 95% efficacy vaccine. You got a silver bullet. The rodent-control people don't have a silver bullet, the hook-and-ladder people don't have a silver bullet, the homicide detectives don't have a silver bullet. You got a silver bullet. But only if you get the silver bullet into arms. Why haven't you shot that bullet into millions of arms by now? How many hours have you been in town? And still standing around looking bewildered among a bunch of files? Why aren't you in motion? Why aren't you out in the field?

So I got in motion. I ran off to the hot red areas on the murder map, the projects and the tenements, and interviewed the families of the recovering measles cases. And it turned out this was Bangladesh in reverse, at least from an immunization standpoint. The so-called "hard to reach" population had been out there in plain sight, banging futilely on the doors of all those primary care clinics that had gotten boarded up because "government isn't the solution, government is the problem." The onerous problem of public clinics in destitute neighborhoods had been solved by boarding them up. Unvaccinated and often sick, the kids and their families had ended up instead at crowded ERs and WIC centers, places where no vaccination was taking place but where they were at high risk to catch measles or transmit it if they already had it.

So we started measles vaccination initiatives at ERs and WIC centers, the most accessible points for interrupting pathogen transmission, acknowledging the potential downside of those improvised efforts was to undermine further the tenuous condition of primary care. About two years later, the outbreak was kicked out of New York City. After a couple more years, through a variety of similar strenuous, improvised efforts in a whole bunch of cities, ongoing measles transmission was stopped in the United States as a whole.

We'd achieved the seemingly impossible, an island of measles elimination in a globe filled with measles disease. And we had done it without waiting for trillion-dollar repairs to the primary care infrastructure. We didn't wait for the rodents to get exterminated or people to stop murdering each other. We targeted our silver bullet with relentless tenacity, and now there wasn't a red area left on the measles map, not even the smallest tache of palest carnation pink. Gone. Everywhere in the United States. Yes, you can say it, even if we're too modest to say so ourselves: we disease-elimination types are pretty slick when we want to be. We published a whole journal supplement modestly celebrating how slick we were. Now our measles elimination story had become part of official CDC history, along with malaria and smallpox.

Whereupon outbreaks began to occur among well-off, well-educated White people choosing *not* to vaccinate their children. We vaccinators had suddenly become nefarious, sinister types, trying to pickle little kids' brains, turn toddlers into autistic zombies. Here we'd thought we were going to be treated as heroes, get carried off on the cheering crowd's shoulders at the head of parade. Instead we find we're under a dark cloud of suspicion, get death threats, have to conceal our home addresses. Easy to cop an attitude. Screw the ingrates. Time to go someplace where the mission can get accomplished with true finality, like the smallpox crew did back in those heroic days in Bangladesh.

So then I arrive in a country where the individual income is less than what American families spend on dog food, where children are dying in the thousands of dysentery, pneumonia, malnutrition. I arrive in the largest city, the capital city, but you're told never to call it the capital city. Awhile back, the previous chief of state decided to relocate the nation's capital from the largest city to his birthplace in the bush where he created a giant ghost town version of Brasilia. It includes a massive basilica that he insisted be a few inches taller than Saint Peter's in Rome, over the opposition of just about everybody, including the local bishops. No one actually works in that empty city. They call it the "political capital," since the vestigial but ceremonially intensive legislature meets there. The city where everybody actually works is now called the "administrative capital."

I'm in the administrative capital on a "consultation." I try to consult with someone in the Ministry of Health. The Ministry doesn't want me there consulting, any more than a U.S. state or locality wants CDC there. Who wants an outsider to tell you everything you're doing wrong? But when most of your funding comes from outside, there's not much choice about inviting CDC. As usual it's hard to meet with anybody. The host country almost always craftily schedules CDC consultancies at the start of a national holiday. And when the holiday's over, the relevant deputy minister is almost always at a conference. Conferences are good. Conferences on any topic, however irrelevant, are very good. You get per diems, travel allowances, free food. You can support yourself just on those conference gleanings alone, particularly since receipt of salary from the Ministry is often uncertain, very uncertain.

I manage to meet the deputy minister at a conference coffee break in one of the big hotels. I tell him that we're concerned that the northern provinces have reported almost no cases at all for the past year. We think there may be more going on there than that. He says we should offer congratulations since that's a disease for which CDC has decided to stamp out the pathogen, has an eradication goal of zero cases. Isn't that why I'm there, to make sure the Ministry ignores all other diseases, all the other causes of death and disability, in favor of that one very uncommon disease that never kills anybody but for which CDC has a goal of zero cases? I ignore the sarcasm. It's nothing new. They say that kind of thing all the time. I persist. I say monthly reports of zero cases might be reassuring. On the other hand, having almost no reports whatsoever for a year isn't quite as reassuring. Ergo, somebody needs to get out there in the northern provinces to see what's going on. That's why I'm here. He gives a big shrug, says I can have a car and driver, but I have to check in beforehand with the World Health Organization (WHO), the United Nations International Children's Emergency Fund (UNICEF), and who knows who else.

I check in with WHO, UNICEF, and who knows who else. They don't want me to go to the northern provinces. They've had it up to here with stamping out pathogens. They're better than us. They're better than CDC. They look after the total health of the populace. They're not just wandering the globe trying to put another notch on the gunstock of some multi-billionaire turned philanthropist who's subsidizing all this because it isn't enough to be filthy rich so he goes looking for some sort of Nobel Prize and mention in the history books as having single-handedly knocked off a mildly disagreeable microbe that never kills anybody. Never kills anybody. Meanwhile, how many millions are dying of other diseases? The historical glory of knocking off one bug, always the historical glory for you greedy guys. You're gluttons for glory. Let's face it, all a typical CDC type like you is going to do in the northern provinces is hijack the infrastructure so it can't lift the total health of the populace, so it can't save lives. Right?

With difficulty I repress what I want to say: you guys are sitting around here in your air-conditioned office in the land of tall buildings, wondering which vintage you should have that night from your wine cellar. All the while, you're spending a bunch of money, more than half of which ultimately comes from the U.S., and what do you have to show for it? Tell me about all this wonderful total health you're producing. Last time I checked, this country was in worst decile of the world in infant mortality. Get back to me when you put just a tiny notch on your own gunstock. On the rate of babies dying.

Fortunately, I don't say that. Particularly since this is all in French and their French is better than mine. Francophones are real good at slicing you to bits. It's their national sport. Instead, I say I'm on their side. Total health is good. Having 54 health indices that you follow from a tall building in the administrative capital is good. Meanwhile, I got a personal problem for which I'd like their sympathetic assistance. My bosses back in Atlanta have sand in their pants over absolutely no reports about their private pet pathogen from the northern provinces for over a year. They're obnoxious that way. All they can think about is that little pet pathogen. Hey, what can any of us do? We all have obnoxious, unreasonable bosses. I'm in a bind here. I don't have a choice. They sent me here to check it out. I can't go home without doing that. You understand. Oh, yes, they do understand. They're not happy. They're going to talk to the Minister himself. They're going to do everything to stop me from going to the northern provinces. In the interest of preventing an eradicationist like me from hijacking the total health of the populace.

I go immediately to the driver that's been assigned to me. He's a big burly fellow. He's seen it all, maybe more than once. We need to leave immediately, I tell him. Let me run upstairs and get my backpack. He shakes his head. Tires will never make it. Those are tough roads. Get new tires, I say. Need money, he says. Get it from the Ministry, I say – the Ministry has gotten a whole bunch of money for fleet maintenance. Never seen that money and never will, he says. There we stand. Out in the heat. How much? I ask. He gives me the price. I say I don't have that. He says I do and leads me several blocks away to a machine in a wall. He nods wisely – you foreigners can always get money out of that machine with that piece of plastic you all carry. I get money out of the machine. He disappears and comes back with new tires on the car. I'm ready to leave. He says the air-conditioning is shot and we'll never survive the northern provinces if that isn't fixed. I go back to the machine in the wall and give him more money. He comes back with the air-conditioning fixed. By that time, it's too late to leave that day. I tell him to pick me up at dawn. He comes by at dawn. He says we can't leave because his family will have nothing to eat while we're gone. He wants his per diems. But that's for him to use on the trip, I say. He gets indignant. How else is his family to survive while he's gone unless he has the per diems up front? Do I want them to starve, wife and three little kids? I go back to the machine in the wall and give him all his per diems up front. He vanishes, I get profoundly worried, those WHO and UNICEF types are bound to intercept me (in the interests of the total health of the populace), while I stand there on the sidewalk nervously pacing up and down alongside my backpack. But, oh what a relief, the driver comes back, and off we go to the northern provinces.

For miles and miles of bumpy dirt roads, I'm nervously looking around, checking the rearview mirrors, till we get out of cell phone range. Then celebration. Yeah, out of reach, catch me if you can! I was the eradication warrior who'd made a daring escape. I was a pathogen-extinction commando inserted into a deep reconnaissance mission. The Secretary will disavow any knowledge...

Things weren't so technicolor when we got to the northern provinces. It was slash-and-burn agriculture, so the tiny cinder block room that I used as my combination bedroom, bathroom, and supreme command operations base was always filled with drifting smoke. Nothing like a desk or a table, but I could sit on the bunk and work. Sporadic electricity, so at night I used my headlamp. The water only came out of the spigot at 4 AM (give or take an hour or so) and lasted only a few minutes, so you leapt from your bed and went rushing about filling every possible receptacle. Then threw lots of iodine in it.

In regard to my bosses' little pet pathogen, it was kind of obvious what was going on, as I made my way from village after village inventorying the situation. In the dry season, the local river dried up into puddles. People put their feet in those puddles and then got their water from those same puddles. So the pathogen had no trouble transmitting. Right there in the puddle was the point of transmission. And there were plenty of cases to go around to transmit. And not much was being done about it. Wellhole pumps lacked handles, and water filters sat unused. Just about any intervention you could name wasn't happening. In truth, lots of bad things came out of those contaminated puddles, not just the pet pathogen, things that killed people, things that killed kids in particular.

However, lack of clean water wasn't the real problem. The real problem was that the northern provinces never saw much of anybody from the southern provinces. The northern provinces were Muslim. The southern provinces were Christian. The southern provinces were where the two capitals were. The northern province folks didn't see much point in reporting anything to the southern provinces if you never saw anybody and never heard anything from them except how big their basilica was. So the whole thing wasn't too tough to figure out. Solving it was a different matter.

So I went back to the administrative capital and installed myself in a cheap guesthouse. The guesthouse was operated by a Brit who was building plank by plank a sailboat with which to travel around the world. I never found out exactly why he came all the way here to do that, but it was a reassuring 19th century touch – there was still an eccentric Englishman high and dry in an obscure corner of the planet, taking tea at Greenwich Mean Time just like in the Victorian days. You felt the continuity of history – the Empire and Pax Britannica. Since I wasn't in the northern provinces anymore, WHO and UNICEF left me alone. I wrote my report in peace and quiet while the Englishman sanded his mizzenmast or whatever it was.

I handed in my report and got on a plane. I didn't learn anything about the local languages, I didn't learn anything about the local cultures, I didn't learn anything about the local history. In short, I was exactly who I was supposed to be. I was from CDC, and we were going after the pathogen at its most accessible point.

But sometimes it's hard to be only who you're supposed to be. In addition to an 18-page report with annexes and tables and bibliography and acknowledgments and executive summary, what I brought back from the northern provinces was a memory of the mudbrick mosques, each a different work of art on its own, with little turrets and crenellations and serpentine decorations, each worthy of being a Gaudí cathedral in miniature, each surrounded by a village's thatch huts, each looking like it'd dissolve like a sand castle in a hard rain, each designed by villagers who couldn't read or write. The passage of time can be a powerful thing. Images linger and grow stronger. Here's one more.

In the evenings, the driver and I would go to the local café, which consisted of nothing but some folding chairs and somebody's charcoal stove. When night fell, the proprietors would crank up the generator, pull out the 13-inch TV, extend the antenna above the thatch roof. Half the village would gather round, and we'd all watch Brazilian soap operas dubbed into French. This was a fully engaged audience – lots of "Don't believe him, he's cheating on you!" or "Don't leave, he didn't mean it!" Once a night, overhead, there'd be the tiny lights of a transcontinental airliner heading from the administrative capital down in the southern provinces, past our northern provinces, up across the Sahara to Europe. From their windows, we probably didn't register as anything but darkness.

There, watching dubbed telenovelas in the invisible café, the tiny lights of that nightly plane seemed sadly pertinent. If you took the view from 30,000 feet, the big view, the total-health-of-the-populace view, you never saw anything, there was no reason to go anywhere, it's all long-distance calls and spreadsheets with 54 critical indices and tall buildings and a sommelier offering an unusual vintage. The northern provinces never hear from the southern provinces, and it goes on forever. On the other hand, if you have a mission, if you're highly focused, even narrow minded about the mission, it's true you can get obsessed, true you can have motivations as contaminated as the water, true you can do all sorts of inadvertent damage in your greed to do good – but at least your feet are held to the fire. Sooner or later, you have to dive into the messy middle of things, see the muddy puddles where people drank their water and got their diseases, see the Gaudí mosques, see the dubbed telenovelas, and then try to understand what's going on, try to do something about it. And you can't do that from 30,000 feet or sitting in an office park cubicle staring at pretty numbers scrolling down a spreadsheet. If you're never out there in the mess, you don't really know what's going on. Your uniform never gets dirty. And you feel nothing.

Shortly after my return, the northern provinces revolted. Civil wars started and stopped and restarted, with France switching sides periodically since its old colony had economic value as a coffee producer. On some coffee basis or another, peace was finally restored, and allegedly the pet pathogen was eradicated from the northern provinces. So maybe some good was done. We'd all like to think that, wouldn't we? About what we do. How else can we be part of the history? Part of something greater than ourselves?

Everybody at CDC has these stories, these tall tales, we've all got a zillion, they're our songbook, you can hear them sung in all the hallways and all the cubicles, across the conference calls and teleconferences, a cacophonous multi-aria opera constantly playing in stairwells and parking lots, through bathroom partitions, next to urinals. Sort of like birds chirping in the trees, we're telling ourselves who we are, what we're doing, what we want to do.

A Japanese physician spent several months at CDC on some sort of exchange program and was placed in a cubicle near mine, so we often chatted. He was summoned back early to Japan to head up some health agency or another there, but he did debrief us on his impressions of CDC. Being a polite fellow, he didn't mention things like our obvious lack of manners, our arrogance in thinking we ruled the planet, our bafflement with people who just couldn't be a little more like us. He said he was most struck by our optimism that any problem could be solved, our unsparing optimism. Clearly a euphemism. You had the sense that for him this unsparing optimism had become an almost oppressive quality, permeating all the stories that we told about ourselves, the history we'd constructed.

Hard to refute. After returning from the field, whether in the States or abroad, we disease-elimination types tend to come back with the same story, the story that we can trust no one but ourselves. Others, those so-called experts, those so-called representatives, those so-called custodians of the public weal, are always trying to stop us. They have selfish motives. Even corrupt motives. We don't. Controversy, fuss, opposition may even be evidence that we're making headway against selfishness and corruption. We're trying to save people. Sometimes even people who don't want to be saved. But we're going to save them anyway. Wars happen, revolts happen, droughts, earthquakes, genocides, assassinations, suicide bombers, plagues, mass migrations, hurricanes. We're not deterred. We're relentlessly tenacious, we have unsparing optimism, we have purity of purpose. We learned our trade in every unpromising corner of the nation and the world, we were sent to those places exactly because they were unpromising, and we got it done. That's our story, that's our history, that's who we are.

Now we're home, back in the office park cubicle or bedroom office, singing our stories all with same refrain, inspiring ourselves with a righteous impatience, an eager readiness to cut corners, an unspoken pissed-off willingness to do whatever it takes to get it done. Yes, now we're going to apply that same incorruptibility, that same unsparing optimism, purity of purpose, nay even fanaticism, to the opioid epidemic that has defeated all others in the past.

Rule #1: Go after the pathogen. Interrupt its transmission at the most accessible point.

PART III

THE VERY BEST LOW-QUALITY SCIENTIFIC DATA

Nothing is easier than for passion to overcome reason. Its greatest triumph is to overcome self-interest.

– Jean de La Bruyère (1645-1696), *Les Caractères,* "Du Coeur," no. 77

They lost sight of their objectives, so they re-doubled their efforts.

– Common conclusion to CDC oral debriefings on ineffective disease-control efforts (by somebody else)

CHAPTER EIGHT

Weaponizing Weakness

On March 18, 2016, CDC published its "Guideline for Prescribing Opioids for Chronic Pain, United States, 2016." A chapter or so ago, you may remember, we left CDC standing idly around while the U.S. consumed 80% of the world's opioids, millions of doses were dumped into rural towns of a couple hundred souls, and overdose rates were on the rise. So this is CDC moving into action.

Moving into action may not be exactly descriptive. In a legal sense, CDC is powerless. It can't tell anybody to do anything. It's not a law enforcement or regulatory agency. The most humble personal injury attorney operating out of a basement has more formal leverage – to issue subpoenas, take testimony under oath, obtain court orders. CDC can do none of that. No one has to talk to us, no one has to listen to us, no one has to do anything we want. Doesn't matter if it's a national emergency. We can't sortie outside of CDC to investigate anything, no matter how imminent the threat. Even if it's across the street from our offices, someone spreading plague right there in the public parking lot while giving us the social finger. We have to be "invited" by the local authorities. Which often takes arm-twisting. CDC can only provide suggestions, produce reports, publish studies, and offer supplemental funding. We only have the power of persuasion. The way we persuade is through guidelines and recommendations. Those flimsy pieces of paper are CDC's weapons of mass persuasion.

It's a rare medical epidemiologist ("med epi") who really wants to work on one of those things. You'd rather do your own studies or get out in the field. Those guideline things take over your whole life. The authors are supposed to be the Subject Matter Experts, the "SMEs." However, you're the Subject Matter Expert, the SME, not because you knew anything about the topic, but because someone upstairs told you that you were an Expert now, so hit that scientific lit search button and start reading. Read, read, read. It's almost entirely a matter of luck if you, or anybody else responsible for the guideline, ever happened to see a person with the condition for which you're the Subject Matter Expert. It may be a clinical guideline telling docs exactly what to do with sick people, but no clinical training or experience is required. Read, read, read, then start to write, write, write. You're an Expert. Write the damn thing. Just do it.

Once you produce the draft guideline, it's amazing how many people from all corners of the federal bureaucracy find that their calling in life is to change everything you wrote, whether they know anything about the topic or not. The draft becomes a total mess of strikeouts, additions, strikeouts of the additions, re-additions to the strikeouts, strikeouts of the strikeouts, rearrangements of paragraphs, inversion of the structure, wholesale substitution of terms, finally imperious demands to start over and do it right. In the process, sentences lose verbs, nouns tumble down after each other like dominos, different sections contradict each other. Meanwhile you have to keep the thousands of scientific citations dutifully following around the constantly changing text – remember, as SME you're required to make the whole thing "evidence based." That's why you did all that reading. You're an SME, aren't you? So start acting like one.

One guideline for which I was temporarily the Subject Matter Expert took 11 years to produce, handed painfully down from med epi to med epi over more than a decade, never quite getting past anonymous but highly connected individuals in Washington. At one point, 48 hours from going public, it was mysteriously pulled by a nameless person said to work for the White House. Nameless because no one would say his or her name – Voldemort-style. A couple years later, with a new Pennsylvania Avenue occupant, the guideline finally got sneakily released, taking advantage of confusion in an administration change-over. Then it largely disappeared from view, as if it had never been. That's what happens when you have good science but no political will whatsoever behind it. No political will, nothing happens. The fate of so many guidelines.

But how about a politically supported guideline? They do exist. For those, at the point of public launch, the authors are relegated to the background, occasionally mentioned but rarely seen or heard. Everyone knows that med epis are famously unable to stay on message, can never seem to remember the five key points Media Relations told them to check off in any response, obliviously imagining that the public is as interested as they are in the fascinating obscurities of the data that they spent so many months and months reading about.

One former CDC Director was refreshingly candid in discussing this vexatious dilemma of dreamily impractical scientists: "There are people at C.D.C. who really don't get it," he told the *New York Times*, throwing up his hands at how often he was confronted with the "in some ways charming, but in some ways problematic, cluelessness on the part of C.D.C. staff that their recommendations, their guidance, their statements could have big implications."

So, if a pesky reporter wants to quote somebody, Media Relations just emails the reporter a carefully composed statement for SME attribution – usually an all-purpose sentence or two, cut and pasted from the last press release, using the customary phrases such as "The number of cases and deaths requires that we act urgently on the basis of science to avoid another grim milestone." Could be leprosy, drownings, cleft palates, sunspots, meteor strikes, slippery floors, algae blooms – same language: we always follow the science to act urgently to avoid another grim milestone. Always.

If a visual media type insists on a talking head, that's when the CDC Director's Office steps in. And, wow, they're quick studies – brief them for 90 seconds, and they can talk for half an hour, with great seeming knowledgeabilty, about the infield fly rule even if they'd never seen a baseball game. Easy – just give them the SOCO (the Single Overriding Communication Objective), and they'll take it from there. Plus those guys have that cool background of the American flag complete with gold lace trim and a false bookcase with the empty spines of expensive-looking reference books glued to the front.

But you do have to move fast, otherwise CDC will get scooped on the evening news (even about its own guideline!) by that frenetic guy with a Brooklyn accent up in Bethesda who never saw a camera he didn't like or an issue for which he didn't have The Authoritative Opinion. What's worse, the public adores him – they don't want to see us, they want to see him, with those cute rimless glasses, chatting with the TV camera like he was back home in Bensonhurst, leaning out the window over the clotheslines to explain something in easy-to-understand lay language to a curious neighbor. There's no competing with that unique Marcus Welby homestyle communication talent, you just got to beat the son of a bitch to the evening news slot.

That doesn't mean the line-level authors are no longer useful. Authors are very, very useful – nay, indispensable. The same way that frontline soldiers are indispensable. Members of the public can get pretty touchy when they feel deprived of something they want, or pressed to do something they don't want to do. In such situations, the authors become the lightning rods. They're the ones with their names and email addresses on the document. For a guideline on which I worked, one author received reams of poison-pen letters, including death threats, another person had her home surrounded by a chanting picket line as she tried to take her children to school, and my own computer was trashed by a zillion email attacks with such heartwarming well-wishes as "I can't wait till you and your children die of cancer." Welcome to public health.

Back to opioids. All things considered, given the complexity of the opioid epidemic and its scientific literature, the CDC Opioid Guideline made obvious sense: Americans were consuming far too many opioids, prescription opioids accounted for a substantial fraction thereof, many users of illicit opioids reported that prescribed opioids had been their gateway to illicit usage and addiction, and then the illegal opioids killed them, more and more each year. There you have it in a nutshell. The gateway to overdose death is wide open. Not a big leap to arrive at a solution. Slam that opioid gateway shut. Interrupt opioid transmission at its primary and most accessible point. Specifically: (1) have as few people prescribed opioids as possible, (2) keep the dose as low as possible, and (3) keep the duration as short as possible. This was simple, this was rational, this was plausible. And what's more, the whole intervention was totally cost-free! (Govspeak translation: no additional Congressional appropriations required.) Get out of the way – we at CDC know how to go after pathogens.

Sounds nice, sounds clean, but were opioid prescription limitations actually going to have any impact on addiction and overdose rates? The couple line-level CDC authors assigned the task of drafting the Opioid Guideline were heroically frank: the quality of evidence for an impact on addiction or overdoses was categorized in formal terms as "low." That meant "the body of evidence has major or numerous deficiencies (or both)."

Perhaps a little exasperated with this particular instance of 'charming cluelessness,' the CDC Director published his own article a few weeks later in the *New England Journal of Medicine,* stating that "the guideline uses the best available scientific data." Not exactly an untruth, if you give the Director the courtesy of italicizing the word "available." Never one to obsess about nuances, the Director concluded by laying it smack on the table, "The science of opioids for chronic pain is clear: for the vast majority of patients, the known, serious, and too-often-fatal risks far outweigh the unproven and transient benefits."

Unmentioned by the Director was a practical advantage to the weakness of evidence. It freed the hands of CDC to designate the prescribing rules it preferred – absent good evidence, it's a judgment call. And this was taken one step further – no evidence of effectiveness was taken as evidence of no effectiveness. If no studies had been done, or the studies provided insufficient data on a topic, then opioids shouldn't be prescribed. This certainly made it easier to limit opioid prescriptions, since effectiveness had not been specifically studied for lots of conditions, lots of diseases, lots of medications, lots of dosages, lots of durations, lots of people.

So CDC leveraged weak data to tell clinicians exactly what they should do. For acute pain, opioids should be prescribed for only 3 days. Or 7 days max under unusual circumstances. For chronic pain (defined as longer than 3 months), the dosage should not exceed the equivalent of 50 milligrams of morphine, and clinicians should "carefully justify" going to 90 milligrams, above which no recommendation exists and hence should not be exceeded. Almost all these dosages limitations were designated Category A, or "applies to all persons." Only a few were designated Category B, or "individual decision making needed." Ingenious: the weaker the evidence, the stronger and broader the recommendation.

In public health, as in politics, you have to seize the moment. And CDC was seizing the moment. At that moment, the opioid overdose toll (pitifully small compared to future numbers) was transiently prime-time stuff, screaming headline material about another grim milestone (remember, our favorite phrase). But any mortality rate that goes on long enough eventually produces fatigue, gets accepted as a fact of life, gets ignored. At some point in the future, the fickle public will forget that yearly toll of 42,000 or so lethal opioid overdoses, get frantically alarmed about an invading virus from abroad (e.g., West Nile from Egypt, MERS from Saudi Arabia, Ebola from Guinea, Zika from Brazil, maybe something from a wet market in Wuhan...), or even start worrying about the much larger contributors to the annual toll of 3 million deaths in the U.S., like the 606,000 from cancer or the 655,000 from heart disease. In public health, it's all a question of limited public bandwidth. Carpe diem. Seize the moment now, with overdoses temporarily in the headlines, so this opioid pathogen can feel the full wrath of CDC.

For the Opioid Guideline issuance, CDC did about as big a public launch as it'd ever done previously in public health. The press release hit the lede hard with a printable quote from the CDC Director himself: "More than 40 Americans die each day from prescription opioid overdoses, we must act now. Overprescribing opioids – largely for chronic pain – is a key driver of America's drug-overdose epidemic." CDC wasn't going to be a loitering bystander while this epidemic erupts: "As part of the U.S. government's urgent response to the epidemic of overdose deaths," the press release went on, "the Centers for Disease Control and Prevention (CDC) today is issuing new recommendations for prescribing opioid medications for chronic pain."

In a joint media conference with the CDC Director, the Secretary of the Department of Health and Human Services (HHS) repeated the SOCO: "The opioid epidemic is one of the most pressing public health issues in the United States today.... The guideline that CDC is releasing today will provide safer pain management while helping us reduce opioid abuse. It's an important step in our work to combat the opioid epidemic." The CDC Director spelled out the goal: "Really what we hope to see is fewer deaths from opiates, all sorts of opiates. Both legal and illegal. That's the bottom line here.... Ultimately, we want to see the number of deaths come down. It's just a horrific fact that we're seeing it continue to increase."

And the media didn't fail to respond, eagerly picking up the theme of an epidemic, with frequent repetition of the key word, "crisis." Under the banner "C.D.C. Painkiller Guidelines Aim to Reduce Addiction Risk," the *New York Times* reported that "in an effort to curb what many consider the worst public health drug crisis in decades, the federal government on Tuesday published the first national standards for prescription painkillers." The *Washington Post* headlined "CDC warns doctors about the dangers of prescribing opioid painkillers, and began, "With no end to the nation's opioid crisis in sight, the federal government on Tuesday issued final recommendations that urge doctors to use more caution...." Under the headline "Doctors told to avoid prescribing opiates for chronic pain," *USA Today* announced that "the CDC's hard line on opiates is a major shift from conventional wisdom about relieving pain." And *The Guardian* explained, "Escalating deaths and addiction rates force agency – which typically leaves drug regulation to the FDA – to make rare decision to step in."

At CDC we rely strictly on persuasion. And sometimes we're not half bad at it. Particularly when we can be seen as acting in a crisis, and there's political will ready-made and ready to go. And in this case, the political will was poised and raring to go. Senator Edward Markey (D-MA) told *USA Today*: "Just as we need rules of the road to prevent injury and death, we need strong guidelines that can help prevent abuse of and addiction to opioid painkillers." Senator Joe Manchin (D-WV) told the *Washington Post,* "I have pushed for the release of these guidelines because I have seen firsthand the devastating effects of prescription drug abuse on individuals, families, and communities." He called the Opioid Guideline "a critical part of our fight to end this epidemic."

This particular guideline was definitely not going to be a publish-and-vanish document, like so many guidelines in so many other fields. The dosage limitations "will not be seen as voluntary" was the unhappy prediction to the *New York Times* by a representative of the Pain Action Alliance, an advocacy group for chronically ill patients. Similar predictions were repeated by representatives of cancer survivors and pain specialist physicians who complained that their input had been ignored in formulating the Guideline.

And, sure enough, the major policymakers in the public and private sectors immediately started falling all over each other in a competition to translate CDC words into concrete action, very concrete action. Mandates. No CDC guideline in memory had ever been implemented this swiftly, this thoroughly, this specifically, and this zealously.

By October 2018, 33 states had passed laws requiring that medical providers conform to some aspect of the CDC Opioid Guideline, with most limiting initial opioid prescriptions to no more than 7 days. At least one state made it illegal to prescribe opioids stronger than the 90 morphine milligram equivalents specified in the Guideline. The same year, a bipartisan bill was introduced in the Senate (though it failed to be enacted) that would have limited all initial opioid prescriptions to the 3 days specified in the Guideline. The Departments of Defense and Veterans Affairs jointly published a set of policies almost identical to the CDC Guideline. In November 2018, Medicare announced reimbursement rules conforming to the CDC Guideline. Similarly, multiple health insurance companies (e.g., Blue Cross, Cigna, United Healthcare) created payment limitations on opioids, often even more restrictive than the CDC Guideline. Not to be outdone, pharmacy chains (e.g., Express Scripts, CVS, Walmart) began implementing their own restrictions consistent with, or even more restrictive than, the CDC Opioid Guideline. By August 2019, 35 out of 50 state Medicaid programs had implemented reimbursement rule changes that reflected dosage recommendations of the Guideline. The Oregon Medicaid program even proposed that all patients with chronic pain have their opioid dosages tapered to zero. Zero. Now we're talking about really interrupting pathogen transmission.

Within two years, opioid prescribing rates had dropped dramatically within key provider groups: primary care clinicians down 40%, cancer specialists down 60%, ER docs down 71%. Merely by our arts of persuasion, the whole country had raced to embrace the simple, rational, plausible, cost-free intervention of opioid prescription limitations – in much the same way that it had previously embraced the simple, rational, plausible intervention of mandatory minimum sentences for drug offenses.

To emphasize that linkage to the criminal justice system, the CDC Chief Deputy Director, the second-in-command, took her turn promoting the new Guideline, this time in a 2017 article in the *Journal of the American Medical Association*. After first reiterating that "the United States is in the midst of an opioid overdose epidemic," she declared proudly that "CDC works with law enforcement to help identify trends in prescribing practices and associated risk factors and direct their efforts to emerging illicit threats. In turn, law enforcement seizure data help various state and federal agencies target high burden areas...."

Not everyone was impressed. Two prominent academic researchers in pain control publicly lamented that the weak data behind the CDC Opioid Guideline had been "weaponized." Two others, equally prominent, complained in the *Journal of the American Medical Association* about the repeated usage of what they considered to be inflammatory and menacing language, as if physicians were prescribing a pathogen to their patients: "No clinician wants to be accused of contributing to the opioid 'epidemic.'" An article in the *Mayo Clinic Proceedings* phrased things in its title still more strongly: "Murder Liability for Prescribing Opioids: A Way Forward?"

CHAPTER NINE

A Comedy of Errors, or Cruel and Inhuman Punishment?

I really liked the Opioid Guideline when it came out. It seemed pretty neat. I was working in a federal Native American health center that was floundering in its efforts to address its own opioids problem. I was happy to have a big document that would give me specific direction on narcotic dosing, about which I knew very little. Maybe there were other opioid guidelines floating around, but I didn't know about them. Still, the whole thing was a little unusual. CDC does public health. It doesn't usually go around telling docs specific dosages for specific clinical conditions unless it's to prevent spread of communicable diseases, like tuberculosis or HIV. And even there, clinical treatment guidelines are issued in collaboration with a whole bunch of clinically oriented medical organizations, or left entirely to the clinical organizations maybe with an *ex officio* CDC rep. I'd sat *ex officio* on one of those panels for development of HIV treatment guidelines and kept my mouth shut to let the people who treat HIV for a living do their thing, my only contribution being to correct a typo or two. In contrast, this Opioid Guideline had no clinical organization collaborators, no academics in the field of pain management as coauthors. Zero. CDC didn't seem to have done any studies of its own out in the field, or outbreak investigations, or anything that suggested they'd ever ventured beyond the numerical simplicity and clarity of randomized controlled trials and metanalyses on a computer screen, out into the grimy, topsy-turvy, unpredictable outside world of actual opioid use.

But why should I care? Here at the Native American health center, we were definitely in the grimy, topsy-turvy, unpredictable world beyond the carefully standardized methods of formal reviews of the scientific literature. For years we'd been handing out opioids right, left, and center, like they were gumdrops. The patients had gotten used to those gumdrops. The patients had started demanding those gumdrops. We really had to do something about this gumdrop opioid prescription problem we'd helped create. And now I had a Guideline to wave around. Encounter a little patient reluctance around narc dosage reductions? Pull out this big official document and point to the relevant passage. A weapon. Now we had a weapon to attack opioid abuse. Who could be against a weapon to attack opioid abuse? I took the Guideline to the health center's pharmacy, we copied the Guideline and got it out to everybody who had anything to do with patients. I was the CDC Opioid Guideline evangelist, the true believer. The opioid gumdrop era was over.

OK, you're right, true believers are notoriously unstable partisans. And sure enough, a few years later, I made a remarkably sudden U-turn in attitude – right when staph was climbing up my leptomeninges and my abscessed C6-C7 vertebrae were fusing and I was screaming into a pillow so as not to wake the neighbors and narcs seemed like the only thing that would keep me from burning for eternity in that lake of fire of which Jonathan Edwards spoke. You're right – now there's a narcissistic, self-centered approach to medicine. My defense? Kind of lame, but no less an authority than Saint Augustine said, "Changing your mind is not the same as inconsistency."

The initial reactions of those with clinical expertise about opioids were more prescient than mine, even if their language was judicious. The chair of the American Medical Association (AMA) Task Force to Reduce Opioid Abuse warned about "the potential effects of strict dosage and duration limits on patient care." Similarly, a professor of neurology at Harvard wrote in the journal *JAMA Neurology* that "concerns may be raised that appropriate access to opioids could be negatively affected by federal guidelines based on admittedly weak data."

Then prominent journals began publishing anecdotes and studies about patients who had attempted suicide and even succeeded because they couldn't handle the pain levels that came with reduced dosages. Among veterans, those discontinued from long-term opioid treatment had doubled overall mortality and a sixfold increase in deaths from suicide or overdose, primarily in the months following discontinuance. A subsequent study of billing records for a broad sample of the U.S. population found a similar pattern. Among persons on Medicaid whose opioid dose was abruptly reduced, a study in one state found a threefold increased risk of suicide.

Then horror stories emerged of Medicaid or insurance companies applying the Guideline dosage limitations to patients dying of cancer. A 2018 survey by the American Cancer Society found that 48% of cancer patients said their physicians had told them that treatment options for pain were now limited by laws, guidelines, or insurance coverage. The number of cancer patients and survivors with opioid prescriptions had decreased by more than half in just two years after the issuance of the CDC Guideline. As many as 50% of cancer patients now were said to have undertreated pain.

Nor was the problem limited to cancer patients. A 2017 online survey of 3,000 chronic pain patients reported that 95% thought that the CDC Opioid Guideline had been harmful, and 84% said they now had more pain and a worse quality of life. A subsequent 2019 survey of pain medicine specialists found that 72% had been required to reduce the quantity or dose of medication they prescribed after issuance of the CDC Guideline. The number of potentially affected persons was not trivial – by one CDC estimate, more than 50 million American adults experience chronic pain and, of these, more than 17 million have "high-impact" chronic pain that limits work and daily life activities.

An academic pain clinician, in an interview with *Clinical Pain Advisor*, asserted that his chronic pain patients were "being presented with three impossible choices: One, you can be totally nonfunctional. Two, you can go out and try to substitute some other form of opioid that would help you function, possibly heroin. Or, you can commit suicide." He described this dilemma as an "abomination." A past president of the American Academy of Pain Medicine described the Guideline as "ill-conceived and frankly very harmful." She went on to say that "too many people have already been a victim of CDC's misguided attempt to address the opioid problem." A commentary in the *Journal of Pain Research* by two academic pain specialists attributed the problems with the Guideline to the closed manner in which it had been drafted: "CDC's invitation for meaningful comment can best be described as somewhere between a charade and a comedy of errors…. Remarkably, the actions of the CDC in the creation and publication of the prescribing guideline appear to violate every single standard that the Institute of Medicine recommended whenever clinical practice guidelines are created."

Thus no surprise when opposition to the CDC Opioid Guideline became organizational, both by patients and physicians. Chronic pain patients demonstrated in front of CDC headquarters. The AMA House of Delegates voted in November 2018 that the CDC Guideline should not be used "in ways that prevent or limit access to opioid analgesia." Furthermore, the AMA delegates voted that "physicians should not be subject to professional discipline, loss of board certification, loss of clinical privileges, criminal prosecution, civil liability, or other penalties or practice limitations solely for prescribing opioids at a quantitative level above the… thresholds found in the CDC Guideline for Prescribing Opioids." Subsequently the AMA president-elect, in an article on the AMA website entitled "How the CDC's opioid prescribing guidance went astray," was quoted as saying that "it will be hard to undo the damage."

In March 2019, a group of 321 health care experts, including three former United States drug czars, wrote to CDC stating that "patients with chronic pain, who are stable and, arguably, benefitting from long-term opioids, face draconian and often rapid involuntary dose reductions. Consequently patients have endured not only unnecessary suffering, but some have turned to suicide or illicit substance use." In May 2019, an interagency task force of the Department of Health and Human Services (HHS) on Pain Management issued a report noting the "unintended consequences that have resulted following the release of the Guidelines in 2016, which are due in part to misapplication or misinterpretation of the Guidelines, including forced tapers and patient abandonment."

Meanwhile a closer look at the relationship between opioid prescription patterns and ODs revealed a strange paradox. Yes, in the first 10 years of this century, opioid overdoses had risen in parallel with the rate of opioid prescribing – as might be expected from big pharma aggressively pushing opioids. Then a curious phenomenon had supervened. The linkage, presumed to be causal, between opioid prescriptions and opioid overdoses uncoupled and reversed. Starting in 2010, opioid prescribing in the nation had gone down continuously every single year. However, during the same period, the number of opioid deaths had gone up continuously every single year, doubling by 2017. The dramatic acceleration of drug overdoses actually coincided with the greatest deceleration of opioid prescribing. The most representative recipient of prescription opioids nationally was a 60-year-old woman with a two-and-a-half-week supply of oral oxycodone or hydrocodone from a pharmacy. In contrast, the most representative person who died of an opioid overdose was a 30-year-old man who injected illicit fentanyl, an opioid 30 to 60 times more powerful than oxycodone or hydrocodone.

A study of "cryptomarkets" (online sellers of illicit opioids) found that implementation of a restriction on prescription hydrocodone was followed by a compensatory increase in illicit sales, primarily of fentanyl, a finding supported by case-control studies of individual patient behavior. As one addiction specialist commented, "No one is taking fewer opioids. I can say that comfortably. They are just getting them from other sources." And modeling studies concluded that reductions in chronic pain prescribing, in the absence of adequate prevention/treatment strategies, would increase the number of total opioid deaths through substitution of more dangerous illicit drugs.

Surveys now indicated that only 20% of primary care physicians would be willing to have a recovering opioid user in their practice and 80% were reluctant to prescribe opioids to their current patients for any reason whatsoever. Among persons who were discontinued from high-dose opioids, the median duration of tapering was now one day. Of those with a documented substance use disorder, fewer than 1% received any medications to treat the disorder after discontinuance. The Food and Drug Administration (FDA) was compelled to come out with a Drug Safety Communication, reiterating that "sudden discontinuation of opioid pain medicines" could cause "serious withdrawal symptoms, uncontrolled pain, psychological distress, and suicide." But to little effect. A major consequence was the creation of opioid treatment "deserts," and it was in these opioid treatment "deserts" that the highest rates of fatal opioid overdoses occurred.

Perhaps the most powerful argument against the CDC Opioid Guideline did not come from patient advocates, pain specialists, professional organizations, data reviews, surveys, or modeling studies. In December 2018, Human Rights Watch, an international organization with staff in 40 countries, best known for exposing torture by totalitarian regimes, published a hundred-page investigative report of the effects of the CDC Opioid Guideline. The report detailed a harrowing series of accounts of persons with undoubted severe chronic pain whose lives had been turned into hell by involuntary opioid dosage reductions or discontinuances prompted by the CDC Opioid Guideline. One provider, who insisted on anonymity, summarized: "It promotes an absolute culture of fear."

Human Rights Watch wrote to CDC asking, "Is the CDC aware that in multiple states, its recommendations have been written into law and/or used by insurers, state medical boards, or other enforcement bodies as a mandate for physicians? Does the CDC believe that this is appropriate?" CDC gave no answer to these questions, merely reiterating in an anonymous response that "the recommendations in the Guideline are voluntary." Voluntary was an unusual choice of adjective, since the Guideline specified that most of its recommendations applied "to all persons" with no "individual decision making needed." Human Rights Watch concluded that the situation could be considered a violation of basic human rights since the United Nations Special Rapporteur on health and torture had specified that "the de facto denial of access to pain relief, if it causes severe pain and suffering, constitutes cruel, inhuman or degrading treatment or punishment."

CHAPTER TEN

The Power of Persuasion

The tidal wave of opposition and negative studies must have been a bit of a shock to those three CDCers down there at the bottom of the bureaucracy who'd been ordered to be Subject Matter Experts so they could spend endless hours dealing with endless edits of endless drafts and ever-proliferating citations of the Opioid Guideline. At CDC, it comes with the territory to be excoriated by individuals with perceived grievances, attacked by tiny groups with intransigent convictions, opposed by professional guilds whose members are miffed that their financial interests have been sullied, raked over the coals by contrarian data mashers all in a lather over your disgraceful lack of perspicacity about some tidbit of analysis, or sent venomous messages by disturbed but anonymous people with strange monikers. Fact of life in public health. Nobody ever went to work at CDC to load up on stock options or put millions in offshore accounts. We leave that to our counterparts in big pharma.

However, quite unusual, perhaps even unprecedented, was the sustained deluge of scientific criticisms and organizational denunciations that the CDC Opioid Guideline provoked. And, on top of all that, to hear that you're accused in a formal report by a major international organization of being something akin to a war criminal? You hear that and you go home at the end of the day in your used Volvo to your modest house, pet your modest black Lab, try to pay attention to your kids who are playing video games instead of overachieving. You call out for Chinese food because you just don't have the morale to start cooking and washing dishes. You sit there, staring at the carpet, waiting for the delivery doorbell to ring, and say to yourself, I donate to those human rights guys.

But no need to fret: this goes beyond the injured sensibilities of the three line-level CDC authors. No, this isn't about the loyal little people anymore. It's about CDC. And the mission. You don't mess with our mission. That's baked into our history. We know our history from the days of nuking DDT all over the South to eliminate malaria, through those late-night smallpox vaccination raids in Bangladesh, all the way down to the present efforts to find the last case of wild polio in a famine-plagued war zone controlled by terrorists. We know how to do tenacity in the face of resistance. They can call it fanaticism, but it's served us well in the past, and it'll serve us well now.

Time for the upper-floor folks to caucus with the Media Relations honchos. Upper-floor guys are pissed. OK, we know you PR guys want us to do warm and fuzzy, butter up the public. But why don't you just let us talk turkey to the public – for once? We're not the Centers for Pain Control. We're the Centers for Disease Control. Turn on the TV – there's an opioid epidemic going on. CDC does epidemics. And we're doing this one with the limited means at our disposal. We can't arrest anybody, we can't sue anybody, we can't subpoena anybody, we can't bankrupt anybody, we can't legislate trillion-dollar programs, we can't even figure out how to get "invited" to the parking lot across the street if a humanity-killer plague were being unleashed there in plain view. All we can do is make suggestions. We made the polite suggestion that docs shouldn't hand out quite so many opioids. It's a legit suggestion, a perfectly obvious suggestion, a simple, rational, plausible suggestion, in fact an absolutely necessary suggestion, and we're not withdrawing that polite suggestion under pressure. Sure, there are going to be pitiful stories. There are always pitiful stories. But CDC isn't backing down on the opioid epidemic, any more than it backed down on malaria or smallpox or polio.

The Media Relations people are smiling sympathetically, like they always do. We're yelling, they're speaking softly. They speak softly till we quiet down. They speak so softly that it's almost whispering, they keep saying their favorite mantra: it's better to convert the opposition than to defeat them. Sigh. Those PR guys always prevail, with smiles and soft whispering. And then they pull out the PowerPoint slides:

➡ Step One: Damage Mitigation.

> ➤ In <u>February 2019</u>, before the Human Rights Watch report gets too embedded in popular consciousness, let's write a letter to the cancer specialists saying *we didn't really mean the Guideline to apply to pain in cancer survivors.* It's OK for cancer specialists to follow their much more charitable pain control guidelines. But only for "select groups of cancer survivors." Don't go whole hog, you oncologists, this isn't a jail break. *Same general thing for persons with sickle cell disease* – the blood specialists can use their own pain guide-lines rather than CDC's. That'll get rid of two categories of

patients for whom the public might have too much sympathy if horrifying stories start being too widely shared. Let's term this a "clarification." Keep all this in a couple nice little personalized letters, that way few outside the cancer and blood specialties will know what's going on. Otherwise everybody and their brother will start demanding a private "clarification" for themselves.

➤ Then in <u>April 2019</u>, have the CDC Director sign a letter to the 321 pain specialists (including those former drug czars) who had complained about the adverse effects of the Guideline. Tell them that *the Guideline "does not endorse mandated or abrupt dose reduction or discontinuation."* Again, no publication by CDC about this "clarification," so it's unclear what the impact of any of this might be. Not to worry – mandates won't get rescinded. How else are we going to get anything done in public health except by mandates?

➤ In <u>September 2019</u>, put together a multiagency committee to *issue recommendations for clinicians on how to taper or discontinue opioids.* No need to have any clinicians or representatives of clinical organizations actually involved, just us docile gov types who follow orders. True, these opioid discontinuance recs will be based on "very low quality of evidence" (those scientists just can't stop being clueless), but what we need here isn't clinical expertise. It's a governmental united front. And bring a halt to that unseemly civil war among agencies that the HHS Pain Management Task Force started, with that snippy talk about the "unintended consequences" of our Guideline.

➡ **Step Two: Charm Offensive.** Put a human face to the whole thing. We can't have the CDC logo turn into the image of a grand inquisitor with red-hot tongs. *Get the little people up front.* They may be clueless by our standards, with their chatter about low-quality data, but they're charming in their naivete, compared to us cynical, been-around-the-block-more-than-once, savvy types. The public likes to sympathize with those charmingly naive scientists, they're disarming, they genuinely want to do good. Genuinely. It radiates from them. They want to do good. The big challenge is to keep them on script.

➤ In June 2019, convince the *New England Journal of Medicine* to do an audio interview with one of the three line-level Guideline authors. *Make sure we have a nice smiling photo, practice a nice soft voice, and above all don't go off script.* Reassure everyone that, in regard to the Guideline, "medical and health policy communities have largely embraced its recommendations" without going into too many specifics since we don't have many specifics. CDC is tenderly aware of concerns about "misapplications" and "misinterpretations" and "misimplementations" by others. But at CDC we're human, you're human, we all want the same thing, we hear you, and we can do this together. Always on script.

➡ **Step Three: Announce Victory.** *Get some sort of data out to indicate that CDC's starting to bend the curve.* Stay aboard for the big win against the opioid epidemic.

➤ In July 2019, trumpet on the CDC website provisional results for OD deaths for 2018, and issue a big press release.

(Time is of the essence, so no need to wait for final data or to publish the findings as an article that might be subject to the usual skeptical scientific critique.) *New York Times* headline: "Drug Overdose Deaths Drop in U.S. for First Time Since 1990." And right there in the lead sentences: "The decline was due almost entirely to a dip in deaths from prescription opioid painkillers, the medicines that set off the epidemic of addiction that has lasted nearly two decades." *The HHS Secretary declares that "we're beginning to win the fight against this crisis."* An academic is quoted as saying, "It looks like there's a light at the end of the tunnel."

➤ True, the fine print isn't quite as reassuring: the overall number of opioid-related overdose deaths only went down a couple hundred out of tens of thousands, while the number associated with illicit fentanyl-type opioids continued to increase. *No need to distract the media with these worrisome little subtrends* – keep those inquisitive folks out of the weeds. Focus them on the big picture. Stick with the headline.

➤ And the headline is: Once again, CDC has nailed it through tenacity, even in the face of short-sighted opposition. True, there may be collateral damage. There's always collateral damage, whether it's using DDT to eliminate malaria or kicking down doors to eradicate smallpox. True, the "best scientific data" may really be of low quality, but that's not The Story. *The Story is: CDC is slamming the opioid prescription gateway shut, interrupting transmission of the opioid pathogen at its most accessible point, and getting control of an epidemic that nobody else could touch.* Check out our history – this is exactly what we've done so many times before with so many epidemics, pushing through resistance to conquer disease. It's who we are, it's what we do. Merely through our power of persuasion, we're bending the curve.

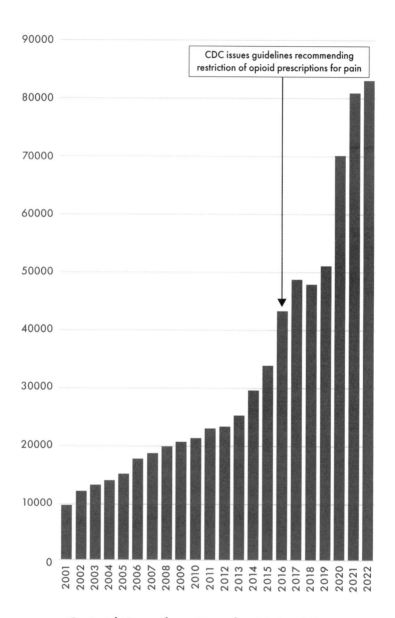

CDC issues guidelines recommending
restriction of opioid prescriptions for pain

Opioid Overdose Deaths, United States

CHAPTER ELEVEN

Bending the Curve

At CDC, we bend the curve pretty often. It's what we're supposed to do, it's what we're funded tens of billions of dollars a year to do, and it's what all us 15,000 CDCers would really like to do. And we do bend the curve in reality. Almost as often as in our press releases.

We particularly like bending the curve of deaths. (Preferably down.) You'd think it wouldn't be too hard to figure out whether we're bending the curve of deaths or not. Death is a binary condition – you're either dead or you aren't. However, assigning a cause to death isn't so simple, especially in regard to overdoses. It's even more problematic if you want to single out a specific drug as responsible. Overdose deaths are subject to lengthy investigation; hence records are often incomplete. Even when data are final, death may be attributed to an overdose but often no drug is specified. And even when the data are final and a drug is specified, more than one drug is involved in a majority of cases. According to one study, the average number of drugs involved in an overdose death was six. A person's death can be associated with a prescription-type opioid, but there is almost never a record of whether the drug was actually prescribed for the person who died, prescribed for someone else and diverted to them, or obtained in some illicit manner. Doubt the complexity? How about Heath Ledger's death from oxycodone, hydrocodone, diazepam, temazepam, alprazolam, and doxylamine? Or Philip Seymour Hoffman's death from heroin, cocaine, benzodiazepines, and amphetamine? So how do you handle all this in public health? As best you can.

From handling the data as best anyone could, it did look like the overdose death toll in 2018 had actually gone down, specifically around prescription-type opioids. Even if it was only by a few hundred among tens of thousands, even if it was within all the uncertainties of the surveillance systems, even if those prescription-type opioids had never actually been prescribed but instead had been obtained illicitly, this was the first time since the 1990s that the rate hadn't gone inexorably upward. In this frustrating, afflicted neck of the woods, you look for successes where you can find them. But then, doggone, no matter what you do, the curve can bend right back on you.

The very next year, 2019, long before Covid got underway, the total number of deaths from overdoses went back up to a new historic high of more than 70,000. Once again, the surge was propelled by the rise in opioid ODs, primarily illicit fentanyl. Then in 2020, as the pandemic really did get underway, overdoses exploded, with a provisional count of total overdose deaths at more than 90,000. And then from every side a blitzkrieg of bad news, almost too much to absorb. More than 10 times as many non-fatal overdoses as fatal ones. In impoverished and minority neighborhoods, a nearly 50% rise in overdose deaths. Blacks aged fifteen to twenty-five years had an 86% increase in overdose deaths compared to the year before. One major city reported three times as many deaths from overdoses as from Covid. The number of pregnant women who died from an overdose had nearly doubled since the year that the CDC Guideline had been issued. Studies suggested that law enforcement closure of pain clinics and busts of drug traffickers were followed almost immediately by a doubled rate of overdoses in the immediate vicinity as pain patients and addicts going through withdrawal desperately sought riskier sources for drugs, a phenomenon termed by the press "the drug bust paradox."

The deeper one drilled, the worse it looked. Naloxone (e.g., Narcan®) is the most effective antidote to opioid overdose – inexpensive, simple to use by the lay public via injection or nasal spray, and rapid in life-saving effect, but the drug needs to be administered rapidly, before the person can go into total arrest. The CDC Opioid Guideline barely mentioned it. And only 20% of persons who died from an overdose actually received naloxone since only a vanishingly small number of people had it at home. By the time emergency personnel arrived, naloxone administration was functionally futile in a person without a pulse. Even among those who were successfully resuscitated, few were sent home from emergency departments with a supply of naloxone – despite the fact that these survivors had a sixfold higher risk of having a subsequent fatal overdose within the next 12 months. Ironically, far more were prescribed sedative medications, benzodiazepines – major cofactors with opioids in causing death by respiratory depression. In the "absolute culture of fear" engendered by CDC's Opioid Guideline, providers seemingly wanted to have as little to do as possible with anything that could be construed by the authorities as aiding and abetting future opioid use – even if it subsequently cost the patient his or her life.

Just before Christmas 2020, CDC put out a health advisory announcing the "Increase in Fatal Drug Overdoses Across the United States Driven by Synthetic Opioids Before and During the Covid-19 Pandemic." It made no mention of CDC's opioid prescription limitations as a method to control the overdose epidemic. It made no mention of the previous predictions of "light at the end of the tunnel."

Regina LaBelle, acting director of the Office of National Drug Control Policy, told the *New York Times*, "We went into Covid with this issue. Rates of overdose were going up; they were on the upswing. Certainly, Covid didn't help and likely exacerbated things, but we were seeing an increase before." Daniel Ciccarone, professor of medicine at the University of California, San Francisco, and the lead scientist for a number of authoritative studies of the opioid epidemic, told the *Times*, "It's huge, it's historic, it's unheard of, unprecedented, and a real shame."

And then it got worse. By the end of 2021, the yearly OD total was estimated at more than 106,000. Opioids overdose deaths had more than doubled since the issuance of the CDC Opioid Guideline. There were now twice as many deaths from overdoses overall as from breast cancer or prostate cancer or colon cancer or leukemia and lymphoma, far more than the deaths from automobiles and firearms combined. Overdoses had become the leading cause of death for those 18 to 45 years old. The total of overdose deaths this century now exceeded the 1.1 million deaths of all the service members in all the wars in U.S. history. By the end of the decade, that overdose death toll was projected to double.

CDC media relations did their level best to put a good spin on all this, issuing a press release proclaiming, "U.S. Overdose Deaths in 2021 Increased Half as Much as in 2020." They made no reference to the new double whammy paradox: exploding opioid overdoses at the same time as nearly inaccessible opioids for pain. Amid the overdose explosion, the opioid prescribing rate had continued to decline, now reaching its lowest point since 1993. Two prominent academic physicians, one from California, the other from Massachusetts, wrote in the *New England Journal of Medicine* about the situation on the ground for clinicians trying to treat patients with opioids:

> Physicians fear losing their medical licenses, being disciplined by their clinics or health care systems, or having to battle every 30 days with health insurers to pay for needed medications.... Today, it is hard to find a clinician who will prescribe opioids for chronic pain – and nearly impossible if you are a patient receiving long-term opioid therapy and seeking a new clinician.... Outcomes include increased use of emergency medical services and opioid-related hospitalizations, increased rates of mental health crises and overdose events, and increased mortality from overdose and suicide.

The addiction expert and noted author Maia Szalavitz began an opinion piece in the *New York Times* on the consequences of the CDC Opioid Prescription Guideline with a simple anecdote:

> Doctors didn't think Brent Slone would survive his gruesome 2011 car crash. His car flipped after he swerved to avoid a stalled vehicle. His spinal cord was compressed. He broke several ribs, a shoulder, and a knee. One lung collapsed. A shattered pelvic bone ruptured his bladder and seriously damaged his spleen, kidney, and colon.

Miraculously, Mr. Slone avoided brain injury. However, he was paralyzed from the waist down. After months of painful physical rehabilitation, he went home to his wife, Sonya Slone, and their 6-year-old daughter. When he had appropriate pain care, Mrs. Slone said, he was able to be a loving and involved father. But in 2017, the clinic he attended cut his pain medications by more than half overnight. He tried to remedy the prescription by calling and even showing up in his wheelchair. Still, he was told he wouldn't receive any refills until an appointment six days away. In agony, he texted Sonya: "they denied script im done love you." He died by suicide in a local park.

Were others as stricken by this simple anecdote as I was? Or was it my all-too-vivid memory of writhing in my bed with staph meningitis, contorted from abscessed and collapsed vertebrae, pleading angrily, futilely, hopelessly over the phone with a pharmacist to release my oxycodone, then letting the receiver drop to the floor and searching my mind for the means to get a gun and blow my brains out or find a way to plummet from a height? "im done love you." There, but for the grace of....

In early February 2022, a bipartisan congressional "Commission on Combating Synthetic Opioid Trafficking" put the same critique in bureaucratic language, detailing the impact on the opioid epidemic and overdoses:

Federal guidelines have focused on reducing supply of prescription medications for acute and chronic pain. Although these well-intended policies have sought to reduce misuse and diversion of prescription opioids, constraints on supply have failed to reduce the number of overdoses.... People with substance-use disorder, unable to continue obtaining prescription drugs, often turned to heroin and then – sometimes unknowingly – to powerful synthetic opioids.... Absent any commensurate increase in OUD [Opioid Use Disorder] treatment, restrictions on prescription opioids have instead coincided with an increase in heroin use and overdose....

The Commission detailed 78 specific actions that were needed. "Without taking these actions," the Commission concluded, "the public response will be unable to stop the rising tide of synthetic opioid overdoses." None mentioned a role for CDC.

All in all – the data, the anecdotes, the studies, the news reports, the opinion pieces, and now (worst of all) that bipartisan congressional report – it was hard to deny there was an optics problem. CDC clearly needed to do something other than issue more press releases about how it was 'winning the fight.' And do that something quickly.

CHAPTER TWELVE

Putting an End to Horrific Facts

One week later, CDC placed in the Federal Register for public comment a revised and updated Opioid Guideline. "Some laws, regulations, and policies that were derived from the 2016 CDC Guideline," the new 2022 Introduction stated, "might have had positive results for some patients." A rather tepid evaluation of benefit, given the gaudy hopes of the Guideline's launch six years before. The new Introduction explained that this was all because of "misapplications." Specifically:

> ....extension of the 2016 CDC Guideline to patient populations not covered in the 2016 CDC Guideline (e.g., cancer and palliative care), opioid tapers and abrupt discontinuation without collaboration with patients, rigid application of opioid dosage thresholds, application of the Guideline's recommendations for opioid use for pain to medications for opioid use disorder treatment (previously referred to as medication assisted treatment), duration limits by insurers and by pharmacies, and patient dismissal and abandonment.

The new Introduction confirmed that the unintended consequences included "untreated and undertreated pain, serious withdrawal symptoms, worsening pain outcomes, psychological distress, overdose, and suicidal ideation and behavior." It emphasized that from now on "acute, subacute, and chronic pain needs to be appropriately and effectively treated independent of whether opioids are part of a treatment regimen." The words "flexible" and "clinical judgment" were repeated over and over on almost every page, as were the phrases "person-centered," "patient-centered," "whole-person."

This was about as strong a seeming mea culpa as any government agency can make. As with most apologies by any agency, this one had to be made by the Guideline's low-level authors, not by the upper-level public figures who had ordered the low-level folks to produce the Guideline. Unlike six years before, no press conferences were held with the Secretary of the Department of Health and Human Services to issue the mea culpa. No dramatic quotes were attributed to the CDC Director. No articles were authored by the Director or Deputy Director in the *New England Journal of Medicine* or the *Journal of the American Medical Association.* Or anywhere else. There were no proclamations about how closely CDC was working with law enforcement authorities around drug busts. No prebriefed politicians gave public endorsements. Just a modest press release expressing modest hopes: "The guideline is intended to be a clinical tool to improve communication between providers and patients and empower them to make informed, patient-centered decisions.... The ultimate goal of this clinical practice guideline is to help people set and achieve their personal goals to reduce their pain and improve their function and quality of life."

Media reaction was equally modest, with headlines and quotes dutifully picking up the theme of the revised Guideline's newly articulated goal of optimizing pain control: "CDC proposes softer guidance on opioid prescriptions" (Associated Press), "Amid backlash from chronic pain sufferers, CDC drops hard thresholds from opioid guidance" (*USA Today*), "In a victory for pain experts, CDC tones down its opioid prescribing guidelines" (*STAT*), "Updated CDC Opioids Guidelines Aim To Strike Better Prescribing Balance" (Kaiser Health News).

The chair of the American Medical Association board of trustees told the *Washington Post*, "For nearly six years, the AMA has urged the CDC to reconsider its problematic guideline on opioid prescriptions that proved devastating for patients with pain. The CDC's new draft guideline – if followed by policymakers, health insurance companies and pharmacy chains – provides a path to remove arbitrary prescribing thresholds, restore balance and support comprehensive, compassionate care." The president of the American Society of Regional Anesthesia and Pain Medicine told the *New York Times*, "It's a total change in the culture from the 2016 guidelines,... a much more caring voice than a policing one, and it's left room to preserve the physician-patient relationship." The executive director of the National Pain Advocacy Center told *Pain News Network,* "I do feel there's some intent to listen to people with pain and their experience, and acknowledge the guideline's flaws. You've got to be grateful to them for that, that they listened. It's a pretty big change for a federal agency." Eight months afterward, validated by this positive response, CDC published the final version of the new Opioid Guideline, essentially unchanged from the draft version.

Even if long overdue, was this finally the CDC Opioid Guideline that might have been – a kinder, gentler approach to relieving pain, even if the evidence level still remained "low" or "very low," even if there wasn't a public rush of insurers, legislatures, agencies, and pharmacies falling all over themselves to relax their rigid opioid restrictions? Three administrations, four or five different appointed or acting CDC Directors, and maybe a little humanity, a little practicality, had finally returned? A cynic might say that it was all just making nice with some aggrieved groups in the run-up to the midterm elections, where control of Congress teetered in the balance. Even if true, what's the matter with doing the right thing?

But there was something just a trifle odd here. In all 167 pages of new Guideline text, the phrase "opioid epidemic" was not mentioned once, the word "crisis" was only mentioned twice, totally unconnected to opioids, and the word "pandemic" was never mentioned at all. Not a single allusion to an overdose problem, not even in the section devoted to "areas in need of additional research." Ditto in the CDC press releases – not a single use of the words "epidemic" or "crisis" or "addiction" or "overdose" or even "death." Zero. Back in 2016, when the original Guideline had been launched with maximal fanfare, those were just about the only terms on the table, and the CDC Director had announced the issuance of the original Opioid Guideline by declaring, "We want to see the number of deaths come down. It's just a horrific fact that we're seeing it continue to increase."

Now in 2022, no press release mention whatsoever of overdose deaths, certainly not the fact that the greatest explosion of opioid overdoses in U.S. history had occurred in the period since the issuance of the original CDC Opioid Guideline. With opioid overdose deaths reaching another all-time high of 83,000 by the end of 2022, annual fentanyl overdoses alone now accounted for more deaths of Americans than the wars in Vietnam, Iraq, and Afghanistan put together. Unmentionable. DEA seemed more impressed than CDC with subsequent trends, sending out an email on May 11, 2023, to all dispensers of controlled substances entitled, "End of Covid Public Health Emergency, Beginning of Opioid."

Did CDC have some secret, unpublicized plan to address the epidemic of overdoses, even though the Division of Overdose Prevention's Guideline, as revised and updated, now scrupulously avoided any allusion to an ever-expanding overdose epidemic? Maybe, but CDC's operating budget for opioid overdose prevention remained unchanged at half a billion dollars, no plans were described anywhere to undo the draconian opioid prescription laws and regulations, and no programs were announced to establish treatment facilities in the opioid treatment deserts where so many fatalities occur. Nothing about how the impact of the new Guideline was going to be assessed. With the "horrific fact" about overdoses suddenly unmentionable, was the Division of Overdose Prevention just going to go out on a street corner and ask a couple random pedestrians if, thanks to the revised CDC Opioid Guideline, those folks now felt more 'empowered as whole persons'?

Hard to avoid the nagging suspicion that there was an unstated subtext here. It was almost as if CDC had wordlessly announced, Hey, we did it. We did what we set out to do, we took care of our piece, the prescription piece, we got pilloried three ways to Sunday for it, we stood up and took the hit for all that, we showed our purity of purpose, we showed our unsparing optimism, we didn't back down, and we pushed opioid prescribing all the way to a 30-year low. A 30-year low! No one thought it could be done, but we drove opioid prescribing right back down to rates that existed long before the Sacklers ever dreamed of OxyContin®, way before big pharma ever collaborated with the Joint Commission to declare that no one could be allowed to have a pain score even a tiny bit above zero.

So what if CNN airs stories detailing how "Chronic pain patients struggle to get opioid prescriptions filled, even as CDC eases guidelines"? So what if, under the headline "They Live in Constant Pain, but Their Doctors Won't Help Them," the *New York Times* reports that "facing a confusing mess of federal and state laws, many physicians are still afraid to prescribe opioids to genuine pain sufferers"? So what if the *Washington Post* and *New York Times* report that state politicians are responding to the overdose epidemic with proposals to "double down" on penalties for possession of minuscule quantities of opioids, e.g., 20 years in prison for possession of a tenth of an ounce of fentanyl in Nevada, three years for a hundredth of an ounce in Alabama? So what if Virginia codifies fentanyl as "weapon of terrorism"? So what if Tennessee charges a 17-year-old girl with homicide since she was the sole survivor of three friends celebrating graduation with some pills given by an unidentified family member (who also died of an overdose)? "Somebody needed to be charged," the prosecutor told the *New York Times*. Now that's called laying down the law: if you teenage girls make the mistake of surviving an OD, you may find yourself on death row.

Not our problem. We at CDC slammed the prescription opioid gateway shut, interrupted the original primary mode of opioid transmission at its most accessible point. And that story is definitely going into our history book, the history we at CDC write about ourselves, right there along with the stories of malaria elimination and smallpox eradication. We did the impossible – we eliminated the Opioid Original Sin.

But now don't expect us to interdict cigar boats offloading shipments at midnight in Florida estuaries or to rummage through the false bottoms of trucks coming into El Paso, or to sniff post office boxes for mailed ziplocks of superpotent carfentanil (the elephant opioid!) ready to overdose a whole state. Last time we checked, there are at least seven different federal agencies that are supposed to be doing that illicit elimination number, hundreds of thousands of beefy guys with guns and some really cute long-eared dogs all tasked to stamp out the illicit opioid variants. We did our licit part. And we just made the licit control part sound warm and fuzzy. Now you do your illicit part. When you get the illicits down to a 30-year low, just like we did with opioid scripts, then we can talk. In the meantime, remember, we don't do horrific facts anymore, you do.

Out in the field, however, far away from sincerely smiling Directors giving earnest talking-point interviews in front of a blue screen background ("What's important to know is..."), far away from any windowless cubicle in any office park in Atlanta, far away from any laptop in a home-office bedroom, far away from any virtual branch meeting with all those tiled faces on mute, out there in the field where no one from CDC ever seems to go anymore, out there where things are always more than a little confused, where the numbers don't always make sense, where right and wrong so often seem to get stood on their heads, out there in the field, horrific facts... well, horrific facts do still happen. Who in their right mind would want to go there? But screw it, why not? Let's go there anyway. And get the uniform dirty.

PART IV

OUT IN THE FIELD

If my uniform doesn't get dirty, I haven't done anything.

– Rickey Henderson (1958-), 2009 Baseball Hall of Fame inductee

Actually my studies involved only the rods and cones of the retina, and in them only the visual pigments. A sadly limited peripheral business, fit for escapists. But it is as though this were a very narrow window through which at a distance, one can only see a crack of light. As one comes closer the view grows wider and wider, until finally looking through the same narrow window one is looking at the universe.

– George Wald (1908-1997), 1967 Nobel laureate in biology

CHAPTER THIRTEEN

Confessions of a Narc Pusher in Appalachia

Let me tell you about my time as a narc pusher in Appalachia. As an opioid pill mill, just two-and-a-half hours from CDC. Or really part of a narc pill mill. A federally financed narc pill mill. And how the transformation of that pill mill might provide some insight into the relationship of prescription narcotics to the opioid epidemic.

There I was, about a year after I'd finished my excursion to the penitentiary, minding my own business in my little CDC cubicle, trying to eliminate some vaccine-preventable diseases in the United States, cranking out statistical programs, and trotting off to try to control outbreaks, publishing my papers, when the U.S. Public Health Service sent out an urgent appeal to docs to help at an Indian Health Service hospital where there was a desperate need for physicians. Memorandum: whenever a desperate need is announced, physicians should run the other way. Apparently I was the only physician who didn't get that memo; thus, I was the only physician who showed up. I installed myself and my backpack in a little bedroom with a bumpy bed in a dilapidated but tolerable reservation house that was filled with clouds of ladybugs and whose common living room had a half-burned log extending halfway across the floor from a cold fireplace.

The hospital, about 200 yards up the hill, looked like a set of bunkers ready to repel incoming rounds – thick cement walls with slit windows set deep in the terrain. You had the sense that those in command had felt surrounded and outnumbered and fled to higher ground for a last stand. The Little Bighorn. The defensive look to the architecture somehow seemed to match the situation. Arrive at 8 AM and the waiting room was already crowded; 5 PM was official clinic closing time, but anybody who got through the doors before they shut had to be seen and treated, so you often didn't leave till after 7 PM. Non-stop complex medical problems: uncontrolled diabetes and hypertension, heart disease and heart failure, lipids out of whack, plus the usual eye abrasions, rashes, falls, pneumonias, hangnails, strep throats, and so on.

Almost all the staff were from the tribe, and at the time there were only two other providers in the clinic, both Native Americans, one a doc, the other a nurse practitioner. They were light-years better than me. And they'd dearly hoped for the arrival of an experienced Indian Health Service clinician and what'd they get? A clinically rusty CDC doc who didn't know the chart system, didn't know what was on the formulary, didn't know how to get an X-Ray, didn't know whom to call over in PT, didn't know how to refer to Ortho, didn't know the number of the lab, didn't know how to ship an acute case over to the ER, didn't know how to do an admission, etc., etc. Three-quarters of being effective in medicine is just knowing how to work the system. Instead of being an asset, I was all thumbs, using up the time of the really useful providers.

But people were understanding. Sometimes it's good just to have another warm body, keep the patient flow going, at least this dude can take a history and do a physical and more or less get things pointed in the right way. And, in fact, slowly I got the hang of the routines. And I really grew to like the tribe. I hadn't worked in a Native American environment before. The working conditions sucked, but the people were great. No one lacked for a sense of humor, no one felt it their obligation to relieve their stresses by imposing them on others. Big sign over the maintenance block: "Fix the problem, not the blame!" It's people who make you happy or unhappy. Fridays, we'd all have fry bread lunch together.

But blame or no blame, there were a couple of striking problems that needed to be fixed. There was absolutely no continuity of care – you saw somebody once, you never saw them again. Nobody had their own doc, nobody had an appointment. The patients just showed up and waited all day and took their chances. And everybody was there for a "med refill." The doc's primary job was to continue whatever care had been started at some point in the past, for some reason, by somebody who wasn't there anymore. And ten, maybe even fifteen, or twenty percent of those med refills included narcs.

I wasn't used to giving out narcs at that rate. I didn't like giving out narcs. I particularly didn't like giving out narcs when I was unclear why they were needed, why a specific dosage was chosen, if there was any plan to get them off the stuff, or if other meds had been tried. Half the time the chart couldn't be found on the big rolling cart containing the charts of everybody who'd signed in at registration. I ended up giving out a whole lot of narcs. Why?

It was just too hard not to do so. You could adjust somebody's insulin, you could go down on their dose of diuretic, you could meddle with their thyroid med, you could stop an antibiotic, but you didn't mess with their narc. The cozy chat you were having in the exam room turned swiftly to confrontation. You'd be told that you didn't know what you were doing, that they'd been renewed on Vicodin every visit for the past three years, that they had ten-over-ten pain, twenty-four-seven, three-sixty-five. Raised voices, stamping out of the room, coming back with relatives from the waiting room to testify that the patient screamed all night, every night of the year. If I wanted to change something, prescribe some Percocet, that'd be OK. Vikes work but Percs are OK too. But if you're going to switch to Percs, don't give me the five-milligram tabs, five doesn't do a thing, ditto for seven-point-five, only the ten works. The ten-milligram Perc. All the relatives nodding in agreement, only the ten works. And none of this every-six-hours business. Needs to be every four hours, only thing that'll hold the pain. And plenty of refills. Jesus, doc, it took me three-and-a-half hours to get in to see you. And I'm all out. The relatives all nod, yes, plenty of refills, that's what the last doc did. Ten milligram Percs every four hours and plenty of refills. That'll work good. The file rack that holds the patients you haven't seen is overflowing, and it's already past lunch hour. You give in, you retain a vestige of imaginary self-respect by insisting on the seven-point-five milligram Percocet. Kind of silly. Nobody comes out of that room satisfied. They didn't get the narc dose they wanted, and I gave out narcs when I really, really didn't want to.

Now, let's say you have one of those rare courageous moments, you consult your professional judgment, you examine your medical ethics, and you don't give in. What's going to happen? You'll never see this patient again, almost certainly they'll keep trying other providers, they'll go to the ER, they'll figure out a way to get an

Ortho or a Rheum referral or some other referral, and sooner or later they'll get the Vikes or the Percs. Narc persistence definitely pays off where there's absolutely no continuity of care.

Or let's say you dig in and really get tough. You write a note in the chart that you were concerned about the possibility of drug-seeking behavior and drug diversion. You recommend that no further opioids be prescribed without a rehab plan, dose taper, pill counts, urine tests. Red note on the front of the chart. Sounded good. A little hitch: there wasn't any rehab program, there wasn't any system to taper carefully or do pill counts and urine tests. All you were really doing was cutting them off cold. Sometimes that worked, but only in the sense that they didn't come back. They disappeared from the system. Dead or alive. You never found out what happened, but your conscience was clean, you hadn't scripted any narcs. That was one scenario.

How about another scenario. Toward the end of the morning clinic, you're actually making progress. Nice woman from admin you haven't seen before, comes in, introduces herself, asks if you could come down to administration, if you had the time, whenever it's convenient, I know you're busy. You didn't have the time, it wasn't convenient, but they were being polite as usual, so you went then and there. The administration was tribal, appointed by the Indian Health Service from members of the tribe. Nice folks, offer me coffee, glad to have me there, everybody likes me, please stay twice as long next time. Meanwhile, doc, to get down to business, I know you're busy back there. Somebody complained to their cousin who's on the Council. They say they'd been on Vicodin forever, all they needed is a refill, and you wouldn't refill it. Doc, please, let me finish, it isn't a problem. Everybody knows everybody else here, so there's no mystery, the cousin on the Council isn't confused and isn't going to do anything, you did the right thing, you were probably the first to do the right thing, keep it up. We got to get ahold of this problem. And because of that I don't want to take up too much of your time, but I got to have some sort of factual account down on paper, just in case things get formal. So if you can give me a little bit of the history and reasoning, I can explain it in case somebody asks me? We need you in the clinic and I don't want to waste your time in a meeting with an elder.

Maybe half an hour later, you head back to the clinic. Meanwhile your patients-to-be-seen rack is completely filled now, the lunch hour is coming to a close, and you just hope there aren't more narc-refill types in that rack. If there are, just sign the damn refill and try to get something to eat before the afternoon rush starts.

You ended up a pill mill. Excuses? Sure, this is back in the good old days when pain scores were the Fifth Vital Sign and OxyContin® wasn't addictive. And no one could say I was initiating narcs – all I was doing was a med refill. I was just continuing what everybody else was doing. Hey, face it, the place is a federally funded pill mill. All I am is a tiny temporary part of it. It will continue being a federally financed pill mill when I am back in my cubicle in Atlanta writing SAS code again for a living. And apropos, let's not lose our numerical objectivity. Numerical objectivity is key in medicine. I was doing good for the other eighty, ninety percent of patients. As for the small minority remaining, the ones who got narcs, maybe half of them really did have all the pain they claimed – ten-over-ten pain, twenty-four hours a day, seven days a week, three-sixty-five days a year.

I could crank the numbers all I wanted, but there was no getting around it: for some five, ten percent, I was a narc pusher. And I hated it. But I couldn't figure out a way not to be a narc pusher.

The tribe figured out a way. They took over the hospital. The hospital had always been entirely staffed by members of the tribe, including all the way up through the administrative level. But the budget was controlled by the federal government, as were most of the critical management decisions since the top staff were all hired and fired by someone in a federal building somewhere in a different state. The potential switch to tribal governance was viewed with some apprehension by the professional staff, some of whom were not tribal members. Soon as the rumors started, people started putting in for transfers to other Indian Health Service facilities. The tribe was a vigorous democracy, elections were coming, and there was no lack of denunciations among opposing candidates for corruption, nepotism, fraud. The tribal newspaper was full of accusations. If you believed a quarter of them, the sky was about to fall, no matter who won.

And the underlying issue wasn't that trivial. A couple years back, after much equivocation, the tribe had decided to have a casino. The casino got built, now revenue was coming in, and the revenue was pretty good. What to do with the revenue? On one side, just distribute all the revenue to every tribe member per capita. Simple and hard to beat as an election promise: vote for me and you're all going to get money, this isn't a promise, it's a guarantee, we're talking real dollars and cents, matter of fact I'll tell you exactly how many dollars and cents you're going to get in your pocket, and all you have to do is vote for me. On the other side, here's the proposition: vote for me and you'll still get a per capita payment, but it'll be half of what you'd otherwise get, and we'll take the rest and go after infrastructure improvements: the hospital, the schools, the penal system. Defying every American materialistic tradition, the tribal members voted to forego getting extra money themselves in favor of improving the infrastructure.

So the hospital became a tribal hospital. The newly elected Principal Chief immediately appointed a young tribal member with an MBA as the new hospital administrator. His first act was to collect as many of the staff as possible and jump on bicycles and pedal the route of a mass expulsion that had taken the larger portion of the tribe to Oklahoma a century and a half before, killing many en route. Pure symbolism. But good symbolism in a context where obesity and diabetes and hypertension were so rampant.

Next, he appointed a talented physician with a degree in industrial engineering as clinical director. The first objective was continuity of care. Every tribal member was given the choice of docs. If they didn't choose a doc, one was assigned. Teams were created where nurse practitioners would see patients with defined problems and the docs would see those for whom a physician seemed to be needed. Visits took place by appointment and were regularly scheduled – no more walk-in chaos. If a patient didn't make an appointment, one was made for them to assure ongoing preventive care. An electronic medical record was instituted so performance on critical health indices could be tracked and the lost chart syndrome could be eliminated. Ten major health indicators were established, primarily around prevention and treatment of the diseases causing the most morbidity and mortality in the tribe. The teams were provided with comparative monthly feedback, with friendly competition producing performance improvements.

To generate more revenue, the electronic record was put to use in extracting insurance reimbursement source, so the hospital needed less and less subsidy from the casino. (To be absolutely truthful, the incessant and intrusive demands of the electronic medical record and the billing system, for all their undoubted benefits, turned out to be royal clerical pains in the ass.) With augmented revenue, the administrator and the chief clinician worked with architects to design a new hospital where patient flow could follow the team primary care approach. That new hospital was built, airy and light and spacious. Instead of needing to send out desperate appeals for help, the hospital became a highly desired environment for physicians. There was lots of competition to get the jobs up there in the beautiful Appalachians.

Narcs didn't get left out. And the policies came from consensus by the providers meeting weekly, with the clinical administrators attending. The ER only gave out scripts with pill counts ample enough only for the patient to see their primary care team, who could follow them on an ongoing basis. A chronic pain clinic was established for those patients for whom opioids needed to be managed long-term, with protocols for dosage tapering and precautions against diversion of narcotics to others. The hospital was connected to an internet-based system to determine what opioids, if any, the patient may have received from pharmacies outside the tribal system. The clinical and pharmacy staff went over the narcotic formulary and reduced it to a minimal number of choices, with expensive and sexy-sounding brand name products eliminated. Teams and individuals were monitored for their opioid prescribing habits, with marked reduction in overall opioid prescription rates, and the total elimination of the med-refill syndrome that had made the old hospital a pill mill.

None of this happened overnight, but I worked in that hospital a couple weeks a year for more than 20 years, so I outlasted most of the medical staff. In some ways, my intermittency may have given me a unique insight into the radical improvement in health care delivery that had occurred slowly and incrementally. Now the place was being used as a positive example for the rest of the nationwide system of health care for Native Americans.

By the end, I found myself sitting in one of the airy, spacious clinics, subbing for a doc on vacation, bored out of my mind. No one to treat. All the patients wanted to see their regular doc and had scheduled their visits to avoid the doc's vacation. And the few patients I did see knew enough not even to raise the question of an opioid prescription. Idleness in a beautiful setting, in a well-oiled system. This gave me an odd nostalgia for the desperate days where, however clumsily, I actually filled a need, treating the malignant hypertensions and the blood sugars of 800 and the fractured navicular bones and the nursemaid's elbows and the ringworms and the rotator cuff impingements and the penicillin rashes, even if the moral cost had been handing out a bunch of narcs. Those days were over. Now it was the opposite problem: nothing for me to do. What was the point of being here? Kind of sad in an upside-down way. It's sad when you're no longer needed.

So that's the tribal medical system picture. But how about the addiction problem? With the end of the hospital being a pill mill, everything must be fine on the opioid side of things for the tribe, right? Not quite. The tribal lands straddle two rural counties that are ground zero for the opioid epidemic. For the seven-year period of 2006-2012, more than 11 million prescription pain pills were delivered in one county (population of 40,000), or cumulatively more than enough to kill everyone by overdose. Almost 4 million were delivered to one pharmacy alone. For the second county (population of 14,000) in the same period, almost 5 million doses were delivered (half to one pharmacy), a cumulative number sufficient to kill all the folks in that county a couple times over. The region was drowning in narcs, legal and illegal. Between 2008 and 2012, the tribal hospital saw a 300% rise in the number of persons with a diagnosed drug-related condition. In 2018, 4,500 persons received that diagnosis in a tribal population of approximately 16,000. The Office of National Drug policy named the tribal lands as a "high intensity drug trafficking area." During a raid in September 2018, 76 persons were arrested and more than $1 million worth of illicit opioids confiscated. The situation may not have been unique to this specific tribe since, overall in the United States by 2020, Native Americans were second only to Blacks in their rate of drug overdose deaths, with only 8% of those who died having previously received treatment for pain and only 11% treatment for substance use/misuse.

The tribal hospital had stopped being a pill mill, exactly as it should have done, and it did so in exemplary fashion. But it hadn't invested as strongly in prevention and treatment programs. No surprise. Same as the rest of the U.S. Cutting down on prescription narcs is cheap. Prevention and treatment have high up-front costs. The tribe had already devoted a substantial amount of its infrastructure funds to medical care. It had equally pressing needs for education, housing, transportation, diversification of its economy. Decisions had to be made.

It's even conceivable that introduction of opioid prescription "best practices" may have contributed to the situation. Let's say you wanted some opioids, for any purpose, pain or addiction. Where are you going to go? Are you going to go to the place where you have to make an appointment (only during weekday working hours), are registered as an opioid-user, twiddle your thumbs in a waiting room, have to fill out questionnaires, may or may not get the dose you want, find yourself sitting through counseling sessions both with the provider and the pharmacist, keep being encouraged to go to group sessions, are urged to taper off entirely, and are put through pill checks and urine tests, with any discrepancy putting you in a thorny situation, maybe cut off entirely? Or, are you going to that friendly guy conveniently located down the road who doesn't bother with any of those time-consuming and annoying procedures, is available all hours of the day and night, and offers you the strong stuff (no underdosing, no tapering here) plus a whole buffet of goodies you can't get at the hospital: meth, coke, roofies, blacks, mollys, bath salts, you name it. That nice guy even extends you credit, and assures you he'll never cut you off, he's your friend, and friends don't do that to friends.

Unlike the rest of the U.S., the tribe figured that out too. In 2018, the tribe opened a $16 million residential treatment center, the old bunker-style hospital converted to a "crisis stabilization unit" where detoxification could be provided. The tribe estimated that it would ultimately need to spend more than $40 million on drug treatment facilities, money that would have to be diverted from addressing other health and infrastructure issues. In an effort to obtain some of those funds, the tribe joined a nationwide lawsuit against the pharmaceutical manufacturers who had flooded their region with opioids.

This last, essential project may represent a fond hope. Opioid settlement litigation has already proven it can drag on for decades, providing full employment for attorneys but considerably less generosity for individual opioid victims. In the tobacco settlement, less than 3% of the awarded $27 billion ended up funding tobacco prevention and cessation. So far, not much reason to think that opioid settlement funds will be treated differently. The *New York Times* reported the results of their 2023 investigation with the headline, "Opioid Settlement Money Is Being Spent on Police Cars and Overtime." A 2024 *Washington Post* investigation demonstrated an even wider scope to the problem of quietly re-directed opioid settlement funding. Such investigations suggest we may need an enlarged definition of the term "Drug Diversion."

The tribe will almost certainly do better. But in an irony typical of such settlement litigation, the reorganized pharmaceutical enterprise previously owned by the Sacklers will only be able to provide funds to the settlement for opioid mitigation to the extent to which the company, as a newly baptized "non-profit," is able to promote and sell OxyContin® and other opioids to the public. Cute: only way to get ongoing funding for treatment of opioid-use disorder will be if more and more opioids are sold. Maybe we'll even see the return of those plush OxyContin® dolls for kids, handed out on street corners as promotions to help keep the local drug treatment clinic open. In the meantime, the multibillionaire Sackler family itself may be immune from fiscal liability, remaining one of the richest families in America.

So the tribe is navigating through a situation inevitably fraught with ironies. In a sense, one can consider all its efforts as a correction for the problem perhaps initiated, or at least amplified, by unrestrained narcotic prescribing during the period in which the federal government ran the hospital. A problem I'd been a part of.

I'll go out on a limb and say (in good, cautious scientific lingo) that the experience of this one tribe may possibly suggest that in an environment where opioids are freely available outside the health care system, the sole use of prescription controls (however desirable in themselves and well-executed in practice) may not be sufficient to reduce overall opioid use. In the absence of treatment and prevention interventions, prescription controls may even redirect some persons into less savory sectors, an unintended adverse outcome that is difficult to quantify from within the health care system itself. These findings are limited by the fact that they arise from a single historical, observational, and largely nonquantitative account, without concurrent controls, based on the report of a highly subjective and biased primary informant who terms himself a former narc pusher in Appalachia. Hence caution is needed in interpreting the results. Nevertheless, the Centers for Disease Control and Prevention may wish to consider whether its Guideline for opioid prescription controls, in the absence of other interventions, is likely to produce an effect on the opioid epidemic that will be free of adverse consequences, intended or unintended.

[Grumpy scientific copy editor: "All OK on those concluding remarks, but suggest avoidance of pejorative terms such as 'less savory' and particularly the characterization of the study's primary informant as a 'former narc pusher in Appalachia.' Doesn't this reduce all chance of credibility to zero?"]

AFTERWORD

There's a funny thing about all of this. Each of us has had severe pain at some point, maybe momentary, say just barking a shin against a coffee table, then hopping around and cursing for a minute or so. But an intriguing aspect of such brief episodes is selective amnesia – as soon as it's over, often you can't remember what it was like. While it was happening, it was all that you were: the cosmos had come to a jolting halt, collapsed onto you, you were incapable of being anything but a pain receptacle. Then it's over. And somehow the episode becomes one more insignificant item in a gray list of unremarkable events slowly disappearing into the past. This is probably a pro-
tective tropism attributable to evo-
lution – you can't keep re-living an intolerable state and reproduce the species. To survive is to forget. But with amnesia comes a certain loss – if you can't remember your own pain, it becomes hard, even impossible, to understand others' pain.

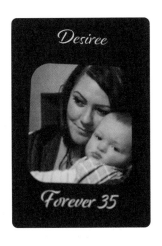

That selective amnesia may lie at the heart of where things have gone wrong with opioids. In a curious twist to human nature that perhaps only Dostoyevsky could understand, we seem to want to punish people who are in pain, perhaps because punishing others helps us forget our own pain – not the pain of knocking into a coffee table but the more seditious psychological pain and discomfort that we can't quite manage to block off and sequester, the pain of our own temptations. Temptations for anything. If we punish others, we don't have to punish ourselves for what we want to do.

The War on Drugs has cumulatively incarcerated millions, destroyed lives, and deprived others of their youth, with no perceptible beneficial impact on drug use or abuse. Unwilling to learn the lesson that medical conditions may not be best treated by punishment, we fell into the trap of expanding that failed punitive strategy into the practice of medicine, with the disastrous consequence of an opioid epidemic pushed to historic highs. What might have been the alternative? Bureaucratically, prosaically, procedurally, it should really have been Public Health 101 for the fresh water admirals at CDC:

1. <u>Don't make clinical policy without involving practicing clinicians.</u> Treating pain and managing addiction are not easy matters. Persons who don't do either shouldn't be dictating to those who do.

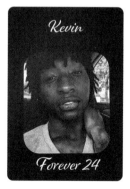
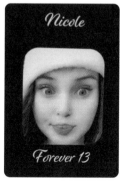
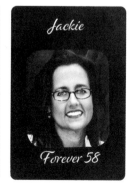

2. <u>Widespread health problems are better addressed by consensus, rather than by edict.</u> The opioid epidemic has been fomented and sustained by many powerful vested interests, legal and illegal. We need all the allies we can get.

3. <u>Exaggerated narratives of fear tend to be counter-productive.</u> The facts of the opioid epidemic are sufficiently troubling that over-interpreting small studies and misrepresenting weak bodies of evidence are undesirable practices, particularly by scientific agency leaders who should know better.

4. <u>Not all problems respond to the same solution.</u> Given the history CDC endlessly recounts to itself and others, it's entirely natural that the opioid epidemic might be seen by CDC as the equivalent of a contagious disease outbreak, for which narcotics are the pathogen. And certainly there are seductive resemblances – person-to-person spread, lethality a function of the size of the inoculum and the underlying health of the host, rapid shifts in pathogen characteristics and transmission systems to escape recognition and control, an epidemic fueled by continual importations, attack rates highest in poor and vulnerable communities, etc. However, even the best-intended efforts to interrupt transmission of the opioid "pathogen" can have perverse consequences, particularly when limited to severely restricting its medical uses. No one ever desperately

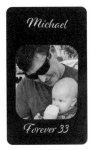
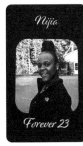
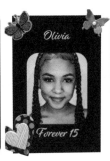
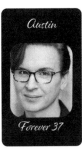

needed a little bit of malaria or smallpox or polio to be spared unrelenting agony or addictive craving. But ignore opioid demand at your peril.

5. <u>Nationwide interventions are best launched after scientific studies have established their effectiveness.</u> The combination of low-quality evidence and stringent mandates is rarely predictive of public health success.

6. <u>Once launched, nationwide interventions need systems to measure both positive and negative effects.</u> When an opioid overdose intervention is followed by the worst surge in opioid overdose cases in U.S. history, the aphorism attributed to Winston Churchill may be relevant: "However beautiful the strategy, you should occasionally look at the results."

7. <u>In public health, you're ultimately responsible for the impact of what you do.</u> If a policy "misapplication" is creating all sorts of havoc, you need to do something about it, rather than trundle out chatter about "empowerment" and "personal goals." In public health, it's never someone else's job to clean up the mess you created.

8. <u>Whatever else you may do, go out and see the thing first-hand.</u> There's a phrase in the military, "If you're disoriented, march to the sound of the guns." In other words, if all else fails, get your ass up to the northern provinces. Or the South Bronx. Or Appalachia.

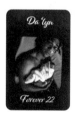 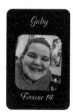 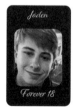 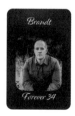 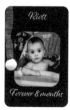

This is all about as plain vanilla as you get in public health. The real oddity is that every single one of those particular standard clichés was ignored when CDC decided to do something about the opioid epidemic – though it never deviated from its central institutional characteristic of relentless, single-minded tenacity in attacking opioid prescriptions (all the while ignoring the outcomes of addiction and overdose). In 2016, the CDC Director, announcing the issuance of the original Opioid Guideline, had promised to go after the 'horrifically increasing number of overdose deaths.' In 2022, CDC's Division of Overdose Prevention contrived to issue a press release about its revised Opioid Guideline without a single mention of the word overdose.

There were options. There are options beyond attacking only one sliver of the problem at the expense of the whole, to narrow greediness. In a very murky situation, only one thing is abundantly clear: interventions that attempt to reduce the supply of opioids, whether prescribed or illegal, without simultaneously reducing demand through treatment and prevention, inevitably

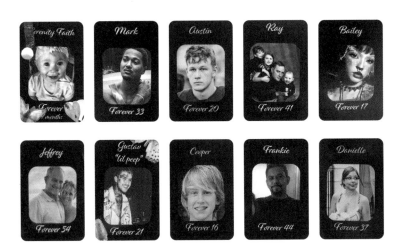

backfire. Fewer than 20% of the estimated 6.1 million persons with opioid-use disorder receive treatment, despite the fact that both its impact and cost-effectiveness compare favorably to the treatment for other chronic diseases, such as diabetes, asthma, and hypertension, where behavioral relapses and remissions are also frequent. We moralize, regulate, and legislate intensely against the dangers of opioids, but comparable annual mortalities, if not worse, are seen for the legal addictions of alcohol (178,000) and smoking (480,000). Opioid misuse holds the distinction of being the medical diagnostic category for which the legal punishments are most severe and treatment is least available. The result is that nearly one-in-ten adults in the United States has a family member who died of an overdose.

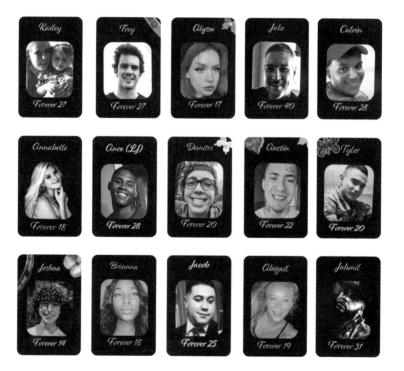

But that's just numbers. No less an authority than Joseph Stalin is said to have remarked, "The death of one man is a tragedy, the death of millions is a statistic." We human beings don't want numbers. We want stories. We need to see the individual persons who suffer and die, with their bad jokes and annoying mannerisms and silly hopes and goofy smiles and moments of unselfconscious elegance. We need to see them as ourselves, as our loved ones. Our policies are

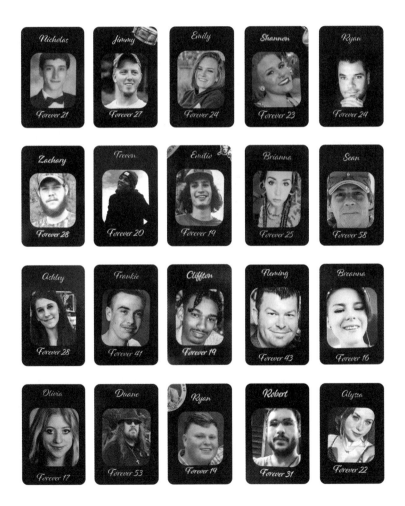

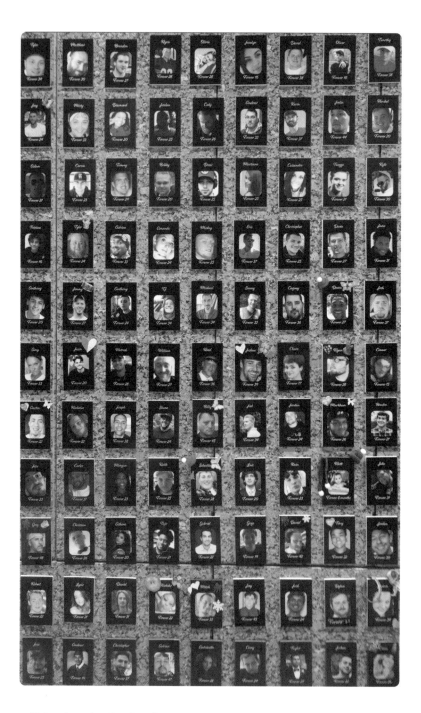

going to be driven by anecdotes that ambush us into an unexpected, even unwonted empathy, an empathy we cannot evade no matter how hard we try.

Whatever specific solutions we ultimately find for the opioid epidemic, the path to those solutions might start with overcoming our selective amnesia – can we remember what it was like to be in inescapable pain, the overwhelming pitilessness of the world in those moments? If we can remember those moments, however briefly, we may be able to escape from our puritanism-pornography dualism, we may be able to recognize that opioids are medications, that they have major uses and major dangers for which a culture of loathing-attraction does nothing but create lethal paradoxes. Perfect approaches may not spring forth in brilliant clarity, they rarely do, but we may be more likely to help, rather than harm, in the messy, emotional, political process of trying to use science to avert death and reduce human torment. We can't bring back to the world of the living the million already dead from overdoses this century, but we can try to stop another million from dying on our watch.

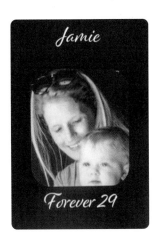

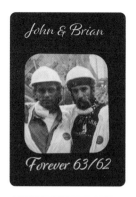

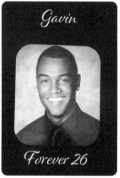

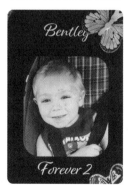

Portraits of a few of the million victims of fatal overdoses remembered by families in the U.S. Drug Enforcement Administration (DEA) public exhibit "Faces of Fentanyl." (www.dea.gov/fentanylawareness)
Photographs of the exhibit by John Canan

Back then, before the Great War, when the incidents reported on these pages took place, it was not yet a matter of indifference whether a person lived or died. If a life was snuffed out from the host of living, another life did not instantly replace it and make people forget the deceased. Instead, a gap remained where he had been, and both the near and distant witnesses of his demise fell silent whenever they saw this gap.... everything that had once existed left its traces, and people lived on memories just as they now live on the ability to forget quickly and emphatically.

– Joseph Roth (1894-1939), *The Radetzky March*

SOURCES

For a prescient account of the prescription opioid issues addressed in this book, readers may wish to consult the January 2019 article by Stefan G. Kertesz and Adam J. Gordon, "A crisis of opioids and the limits of prescription control: United States" in the journal *Addiction* (2019; 114:169-180). The role of illicit opioids is examined in greater detail by Daniel Ciccarone in his September 2019 article "The triple wave epidemic: Supply and demand drivers of the US opioid overdose crisis" in the *International Journal of Drug Policy* (2019; 71:183-188). The human consequences for people in pain are described so touchingly in the *New York Times* columns of Maia Szalavitz (e.g., "What the Opioid Crisis Took From People in Pain." 7-Mar-2022). A first-person physician's account of how easy it is to prescribe lethal doses of opioids but how hard it is to prescribe preventive medications is provided by Elisabeth Poorman in her May 2021 opinion piece in the *New England Journal of Medicine* (2021; 384:1783-1784) "The Number Needed to Prescribe – What Would It Take To Expand Access to Buprenorphine?" Wider matters of public health policy are addressed in Nancy Leys Stepan's book *Eradication – Ridding the World of Diseases Forever?* (Ithaca, NY: Cornell University Press; 2011).

For those who find that facts and numbers alone are rarely

sufficient to grasp, however fleetingly, the nature of pain and death, I suggest taking a look at the beautiful and heart-piercing poetry of Anya Krugovoy Silver who died of metastatic breast cancer in 2018 at the age of 49. It would not be a mistake to start with her final work *Second Bloom* (Eugene, OR: Cascade Books. Wipf and Stock Publishers; 2017) and work backward through time.

Foreword

Opioid Deaths – See references for Chapters Eleven and Twelve.

Chapter One – The North Korean Candidate

Staphylococcus Meningitis

Aguilar J, Urday-Cornejo V, Donabedian S, Perri M, Tibbetts R, Zervos M. *Staphylococcus aureus* meningitis – case series and literature review. *Medicine.* 2010; 89:117-125.

Pedersen M, Benfield TL, Skinjoej P, Jensen AG. Haematogenous *Staphylococcus aureus* meningitis. A 10-year nationwide study of 96 cases. *BMC Infect Dis.* 2006; 6:49. doi.org/10.1186/1471-2334-6-49

Chapter Two – The Fugitive in the Abyss

Shingles Pain

Johnson RW. Consequences and management of pain in herpes zoster. *J Infect Dis.* 2002; 186(Suppl 1): S83-90.

Pickering G, Leplege A. Herpes Zoster Pain, Postherpetic neuralgia, and the quality of life in the elderly. *Pain Pract.* 2011; 11(4):397-402.

Offit PA. Shingrix: Is the Hype Justified? Medscape.com website. 13-Feb-2018. (Accessed 27-Aug-2019).

Poetry of Anya Krugovoy Silver

Sandomir R. "Anya Krugovoy Silver, Poetic Voice on Mortality, Dies at 49." *New York Times.* 10-Aug-2018. (Accessed 25-Aug-2019).

Silver, Anya Krugovoy. *Second Bloom.* Eugene OR: Cascade Books. Wipf and Stock Publishers; 2017.

Chapter Three – Puritanism and Pornography

Nonopioid Pain Drugs: Pain Control Ceilings and Contraindications
Nonopioid Drugs for Pain. *The Medical Letter on Drugs and Therapeutics*. 7-Mar-2022. 2022; 64(1645):33-40.

Prescription Opioids and Risk of Addiction or Overdose – Selected Studies

Hojsted J, Sjogren P. Addiction to opiates in chronic pain patients: a literature review. *Eur J Pain*. 2007; 11(5):490-518.

Fishbain DA, Cole B, Lewis J, Rosomoff HL, Rosomoff RS. What percentage of chronic nonmalignant pain patients exposed to chronic opioid analgesic therapy develop abuse/addiction and/or aberrant drug-related behaviors? A structured evidence-based review. *Pain Med*. 2008; 9:444-459.

Bohnert ASB, Valenstein M, Bair MJ, Ganoczy D, McCarthy JF, Ilgen MA, et al. Association Between Opioid Prescribing Patterns and Opioid Overdose-Related Deaths. *J Am Med Assoc*. 2011; 305(13):1315-1321.

Muhuri PK, Gfroerer JC, Davies MC. Associations of nonmedical pain reliever use and initiation of heroin use in the United States. Substance Abuse and Mental Health Services Administration, Center for Behavioral Health Statistics and Quality. CBHSQ Data Review, August 2013. SAMHSA.gov website. Aug-2013. (Accessed 25-Aug-2019).

Zedler B, Xie L, Wang L, Joyce A, Vick C, Kariburyo F, et al. Risk Factors for Serious Prescription Opioid-Related Toxicity or Overdose among Veterans Health Administration Patients. *Pain Med*. 2014; 15:1911-1929.

Edlund MJ, Martin BC, Russo JE, Devries A, Brennan Braden J, Sullivan MD. The role of opioid prescription in incident opioid abuse and dependence among individuals with chronic non-cancer pain: the role of opioid prescription. *Clin J Pain*. 2014; 30(7):557-564.

Kaplovich E, Gomes T, Camacho X, Dhall IA, Mamdani MM, Juurlink DN. Sex differences in dose escalation and overdose death during chronic opioid therapy: a population-based cohort study. *PLoS One*. 2015; 10(8):e0134550.

Quinn PD, Hur K, Chang Z, Krebs EE, Bair MJ, Scott EL, et al. Incident and Long-Term Opioid Therapy among Patients with Psychiatric Conditions and Medications: A National Study of Commercial Healthcare Claims. *Pain*. 2017; 158(1):140-148.

Shah A, Hayes CJ, Martin BC. Characteristics of initial prescription episodes and likelihood of long-term opioid use – United States, 2006-2015. *MMWR Morb Mortal Wkly Rep*. 2017; 66(10):265-269.

Ghertner R, Groves L. The Opioid Crisis and Economic Opportunity: Geographic and Economic Trends. ASPE Research Brief. Revised 11-Sep-2018. Office of the Assistant Secretary for Planning and Evaluation. U.S. Department of Health and Human Services. ASPE.HHS.gov website. 11-Sep-2018. (Accessed 10-Sep-2019).

Prescription Opioids and Risk of Addiction – Anecdotes
Doe J. "My Story: How One Percocet Prescription Triggered My Addiction." *J Med Toxicol.* 2012; 8:327-330.
Cahoon L, Cox L, Chitale R. "Celebrity Addictions: Painkillers and Hollywood." ABC News.com website. 22-Feb-2008. (Accessed 27-Jun-2023).
Yagoda M. "'There Was a Lot of Pain': 23 Stars on Their Experiences with Addiction." People.com website. 5-Sep-2019. (Accessed 7-Sep-2019).

CDC Director on Prescription Opioids and Risk of Addiction
Teegardin C. "Overprescribed. Healers or dealers? Doctors and the opioid crisis: an AJC national investigation." *Atlanta Journal Constitution.* 4-Dec-2017. (Accessed 27-Jun-2023).

Questionnaires to Evaluate Risk of Addiction Among Those Taking Opioids
Webster LR, Webster RM. Predicting aberrant behaviors in opioid-treated patients: preliminary validation of the opioid risk tool. *Pain Med.* 2005; 6(6):432-442.
Akbik H, Butler SF, Budman SH, Fernandez K, Katz NP, Jamison RN. Validation and clinical application of the screener and opioid assessment for patients with pain (SOAPP). *J Pain Symptom Manage.* 2006; 32(3):287-293.
Jones T, Moore T, Levy JL, Daffron S, Browder JH, Allen L, et al. A comparison of various risk screening methods in predicting discharge from opioid treatment. *Clin J Pain.* 2012; 28(2):93-100.
Jones T, Schmidt M, Moore T. Further validation of an opioid risk assessment tool: The Brief Risk Questionnaire. *Ann Psychiatry Ment Health.* 2015; 3(3):1032.

Chapter Four – The Night Shift Nurse and the Subject Matter Experts

News Reports of Actions Against Physicians Who Prescribe Opioids
Teegardin C. "Overprescribed. Healers or dealers? Doctors and the opioid crisis: an AJC national investigation." *Atlanta Journal Constitution.* 4-Dec-2017. (Accessed 27-Jun-2023).
Teegardin C. "Opioid prescriptions now require database check." *Atlanta Journal Constitution.* 29-Jun-2018. (Accessed 25-Aug-2019).

Rankin B. "Prosecutors notify 30 doctors about excessive opioid prescriptions." *Atlanta Journal Constitution.* 5-Oct-2018. (Accessed 25-Aug-2020).

Berard Y. "More than 1,000 doctors violating state opioid law." *Atlanta Journal Constitution.* 8-Nov-2018. (Accessed 25-Aug-2019).

Kessler A, Cohen E, Grise K. "CNN Exclusive: The more opioids doctors prescribe, the more money they make." CNN.com website. 12-Mar-2018. (Accessed 4-Sep-2019).

"Justice Department charges 601 people, including doctors, in opioid abuse crackdown." CNBC.com website. 29-Jun-2018. (Accessed 4-Sep-2019).

Warren B. "Doctors who fear being arrested for treating pain to get unusual help." *Louisville Courier Journal.* 3-Aug-2018. (Accessed 4-Sep-2019).

Pseudoaddiction
Weissman DE, Haddox JD. Opioid pseudoaddiction – an iatrogenic syndrome. *Pain.* 1989; 36(3):363-366.

Greene MS, Chambers RA. Pseudoaddiction: Fact or Fiction? An Investigation of the Medical Literature. *Curr Addict Rep.* 2015; 2(4):310-317.

Antibiotic Overuse and Antibiotic Resistance
Centers for Disease Control and Prevention. Antibiotic Resistance Threats in the United States, 2019. Atlanta, GA: U.S. Department of Health and Human Services, CDC.gov website. 13-Nov-2019. (Accessed 13-Jul-2021).

"No progress seen in reducing antibiotics among outpatients – overuse contributes to drug-resistant infections, excess costs." Science Daily.com website. 8-Mar-2018. (Accessed 30-Aug-2019).

Durkin MJ, Jafarzadeh SR, Hsueh K, Sallah YH, Munshi KD, Henderson RR, Fraser VJ. Outpatient Antibiotic Prescription Trends in the United States: A National Cohort Study. *Infect Control Hosp Epidemiol.* 2018; 39(5):584-589.

Ray MJ, Tallman GB, Bearden DT, Elman MR, McGregor JC. Antibiotic prescribing without documented indication in ambulatory care clinics: national cross sectional study. *BMJ.* 2019; 367:L6461.

DEA Rules on Narcotic "Abandonment"
Diversion Control Division, Drug Enforcement Administration. Disposal and/or Destruction Q&A. DEA Diversion.gov website. 13-Jun-2023. (Accessed 25-Jun-2023).

Chapter Five – Breaking Into Prison

Incarceration Numbers
Sentencing Project. Growth in Mass Incarceration. Sentencing Project.org website. [No date]. (Accessed 17-Jul-2021).

Individual Incarceration Costs
Vera Institute of Justice. The Price of Prisons. Vera.org website. May-2017. (Accessed 24-Aug-2019).

Cost of Mass Incarceration
Wagner P, Rabuy B. Following the Money of Mass Incarceration. Prison Policy Initiative.org website. 25-Jan-2017. (Accessed 13-Jul-2021).

Prison Spending Increases
National Association for the Advancement of Colored People. Criminal Justice Fact Sheet. NAACP.org website. 2023. (Accessed 27-Jun-2023).

Lifetime Risk of Incarceration by Race
Prison Policy Initiative. Lifetime Chance of Being Sent to Prison At Current U.S. Incarceration Rates. Prison Policy Initiative.org website. 2023. (Accessed 27-Jun-2023).

Local Prison Conditions
Cook R. "Inmates leave Atlanta prison camp, buy contraband, sneak back in." *Atlanta Journal Constitution*. 8-Feb-2017. (Accessed 17-Jul-2021).

Cook R. "Jailbreak! Atlanta inmates escape, sneak back in." *Atlanta Journal Constitution*. 10-Feb-2017. (Accessed 17-Jul-2021).

Cook R. "Boozy New Year's Eve party inside Atlanta's federal pen proves security still a problem." *Atlanta Journal Constitution*. 29-Jan-2018. (Accessed 17-Jul-2021).

Cook R, Foreman L. "From inside prison, federal inmate boasts on Facebook about killing." *Atlanta Journal Constitution*. 1-Feb-2018. (Accessed 17-Jul-2021).

Sharpe J. "Inmate escaped Atlanta prison camp 'for love' – then sneaked back in." *Atlanta Journal Constitution*. 28-Sep-2018. (Accessed 17-Jul-2021).

Rankin B. "Three sentenced to death in Georgia await federal executions." *Atlanta Journal Constitution*. 25-Jul-2019. (Accessed 17-Jul-2021).

Boone C. "Atlanta federal pen nearly vacant amid corruption investigation." *Atlanta Journal Constitution*. 21-Aug-2021. (Accessed 1-Sep-2021).

Burns AS. "Prison officer indicted in smuggling scheme never met co-defendants, lawyer says." *Atlanta Journal Constitution*. 22-Dec-2021. (Accessed 27-Jun-2023).

Thrush G. "Prison Personnel Describe Horrific Conditions, and Cover-Up, at Atlanta Prison." *New York Times*. 26-July-2022. (Accessed 1-Aug-2022).

Corson P. "The Atlanta Federal Penitentiary's Hollywood connections." *Atlanta Journal Constitution*. 28-Jul-2022. (Accessed 1-Aug-2022).

Jackson D. "More people died in Atlanta penitentiary than any prison in the US, report finds." *Atlanta Journal Constitution.* 16-Feb-2024. (Accesed 9-Mar-2024).

Chapter Six – A Beginner's Guide to Kick-Starting an Epidemic

Histories of the Opioid Epidemic in the First Two Decades of the 21st Century

Kertesz SG, Gordon AJ. A crisis of opioids and the limits of prescription control: United States. *Addiction.* 2019; 114:169-180.

Ciccarone D. The triple wave epidemic: Supply and demand drivers of the US opioid overdose crisis. *Int J Drug Policy.* 2019; 71:183-188.

Pain as "Fifth Vital Sign"

Moghe S. "Opioid history: from 'wonder drug' to abuse epidemic." CNN.com website. 14-Oct-2016. (Accessed 12-Jul-2021).

Joint Commission's Pain Assessment Requirement

Baker DW. History of the Joint Commission's Pain Standards: lessons for today's prescription opioid epidemic. *J Am Med Assoc.* 2017; 317(11):1117-1118.

Baker DW. The Joint Commission's Pain Standards: origins and evolution. Oakbrook Terrace, IL: The Joint Commission; 2017.

Prescription Opioids – Types and Prices

Opioids for Pain. *The Medical Letter on Drugs and Therapeutics.* 12-Dec-2022. 2022; 64(1665):193-200.

Effect of Opioid Abuse Deterrent Reformulation

Cicero TJ, Ellis MS. Effect of Abuse-Deterrent Formulation of OxyContin. *N Engl J Med.* 2012; 367(2):187-189.

Promotion of Opioid Use By Pharmaceutical Companies

Van Zee A. The promotion and marketing of OxyContin: commercial triumph, public health tragedy. *Am J Public Health.* 2009; 99(2):221-227.

Horwitz S, Higham S, Bennett D, Kornfield M. "SELL BABY SELL: unsealed documents in opioids lawsuit reveal inner workings of industry's marketing machine." *Washington Post.* 6-Dec-2019. (Accessed 13-Jul-2021).

Emanuel G, Thomas K. "Top Executives of Insys, an Opioid Company, Are Found Guilty of Racketeering." *New York Times.* 30-Dec-2019. (Accessed 25-Oct-2021).

Hoffman J. "Big Pharmacy Chains Also Fed the Opioid Epidemic, Court Filing Says." *New York Times.* 27-May-2020. (Accessed 13-Jul-2021).

Hughes E. *The Hard Sell: Crime and Punishment at an Opioid Startup.* New York: Doubleday; 2022.

Kornfield M, Higham S, Rich S. "Inside the sales machine of the 'kingpin' of opioid makers." *Washington Post.* 10-May-2022. (Accessed 13-May-2022).

Hamby C, Forsythe M. "Behind the Scenes, McKinsey Guided Companies at the Center of the Opioid Crisis." *New York Times.* 29-Jun-2022. (Accessed 2-Jul-2022).

Patient Satisfaction Scores and Opioid Prescription Use

Sites BD, Harrison J, Herrick MD, Masaracchia MM, Beach ML, Davis MA. Prescription opioid use and satisfaction with care among adults with musculoskeletal conditions. *Ann Fam Med.* 2018; 16(1):6-13.

Opioid Prescriptions, Misuse, and Overdoses

Centers for Disease Control and Prevention. 2018 Annual Surveillance Report of Drug-Related Risks and Outcomes – United States. Surveillance Special Report. Centers for Disease Control and Prevention, U.S. Department of Health and Human Services. CDC.gov website. 31-Aug-2018. (Accessed 26-Aug-2019).

Kenan K, Mack K, Paulozzi L. Trends in prescriptions for oxycodone and other commonly used opioids in the United States, 2000-2009. *Open Med.* 2012; 6(2):e41-47.

Substance Abuse and Mental Health Services Administration. Opioid Misuse Increases Among Older Adults. SAMHSA.gov website. 25-Jul-2017. (Accessed 7-Sep-2019).

Paulozzi LJ, Jones CM, Mack KA, Rudd RA. Vital Signs: Overdoses of Prescription Opioid Pain Relievers – United States, 1999-2008. *MMWR Morb Mortal Wkly Rep.* 2011; 60(43):1487-1492.

Number of Persons Reporting Opioid Use, Misuse, or Addiction

Substance Abuse and Mental Health Services Administration. Results from the 2018 National Survey on Drug Use and Health (HHS Publication No. PEP19 5068, NSDUH Series H 54). Assistant Secretary's Presentation. Center for Behavioral Health Statistics and Quality, Substance Abuse and Mental Health Services Administration. Rockville, MD. SAMHSA.gov website. [No date]. (Accessed 8-Sep-2019).

Griesler PC, Hu M-C, Wall M, Kandel DB. Assessment of Prescription Opioid Medical Use and Misuse Among Parents and Their Adolescent Offspring in the US. *JAMA Netw Open.* 2021; 4(1):e2031073.

Neonatal Opioid Abstinence/Withdrawal Rates

Hirai AH, Ko JY, Owens PL, Stocks C, Patrick SW. Neonatal Abstinence Syndrome and Maternal Opioid-Related Diagnoses in the US, 2010-2017. *J Am Med Assoc.* 2021; 325(2):146-155.

Comparison of U.S. Opioid Prescribing Practices with Other Countries

Burden M, Keniston A, Wallace MA, Busse JW, Casademont J, Chadaga SR, et al. Opioid Utilization and Perception of Pain Control in Hospitalized Patients: A Cross-Sectional Study of 11 Sites in 8 Countries. *J Hosp Med.* 2019; 14(12):737-745.

Kaafarani HMA, Han K, El Moheb M, Kongkaewpaison N, Jia Z, El Hechi MW, et al. Opioids After Surgery in the United States Versus the Rest of the World. *Ann Surg.* 2020; 272:879-886.

El Moheb M, Mokhari A, Han K, van Erp I, Kongkaewpaison N, Jia Z, et al. Pain or No Pain, We Will Give You Opioids: Relationship Between Number of Opioid Pills Prescribed and Severity of Pain after Operation in US vs Non-US Patients. *J Am Coll Surg.* 2020; 231(6):639-648.

Opioid Prescribing Patterns After Non-Fatal Overdose

Larochelle MR, Liebschutz JM, Zhang F, Ross-Degnan D, Wharam JF. Opioid Prescribing After Nonfatal Overdose and Association With Repeated Overdose: A Cohort Study. *Ann Intern Med.* 2016; 164:1-9.

Total Opioid Consumption: U.S. Compared with the Rest of the World

Manchikanti L, Fellows B, Ailinani H, Pampati V. Therapeutic Use, Abuse and Nonmedical Use of Opioids: A Ten-Year Perspective. *Pain Physician.* 2010; 13:401-435.

Opioids Distributed in U.S.

Higham S, Horwitz S, Rich S. "76 billion opioid pills: newly released federal data unmasks the epidemic." *Washington Post.* 16-Jul-2019. (Accessed 25-Aug-2019).

Rich S, Higham S, Horwitz S. "More than 100 billion pain pills saturated the nation over nine years." *Washington Post.* 14-Jan-2020. (Accessed 15-Jan-2020).

"Drilling into DEA's pain pill database." *Washington Post.* 21-Jul-2019. (Accessed 25-Aug-2019).

West Virginia Towns' Receipt of Opioids

Eyre E. "Drug firms poured 780M painkillers into WV amid rise of overdoses." *Charleston Gazette-Mail.* 17-Dec-2016. (Accessed 13-Jul-2021).

Eyre E. "Suspicious drug orders never enforced by state." *Charleston Gazette-Mail.* 18-Dec-2016. (Accessed 13-Jul-2021).

Eyre E. "Drug firms shipped 20.8M pain pills to WV town with 2,900 people." *Charleston Gazette-Mail.* 29-Jan-2018. (Accessed 13-Jul-2021).

Eyre, E. "Drug firm poured 3M opioids into WV town in just 10 months, report says." *Charleston Gazette-Mail.* 19-Dec-2018. (Accessed 13-Jul-2021).

Public Trust in CDC

Pew Research Center. "Trust in Government Nears Record Low, But Most Federal Agencies Are Viewed Favorably." Pew Research Center.org website. 18-Oct-2013. (Accessed 27-Jun-2023).

Kowitt SD, Schmidt AM, Hannan A, Goldstein AO. Awareness and trust of the FDA and CDC: Results from a national sample of US adults and adolescents. *PLoS One.* 2017; 12(5):e0177546.

Robert Wood Johnson Foundation. The Public's Perspective on the United States Public Health System. Robert Wood Johnson Foundation (RWJF.org) website. 13-May-2021. (Accessed 27-Jun-2023).

Chapter Seven – Purity of Purpose and Unsparing Optimism

CDC History

Centers for Disease Control and Prevention. Our History – Our Story. CDC.gov website. 19-Apr-2023. (Accessed 10-Jun-2023).

Wikipedia. Centers for Disease Control and Prevention. Wikipedia.org website. 26-Jun-2021. (Accessed 13-Jul-2021).

CDC's Malaria Elimination Campaign

Centers for Disease Control and Prevention. Elimination of Malaria in the United States (1947-1951). CDC.gov website. 23-Jul-2018. (Accessed 26-Aug-2019).

Lisansky E. The Eradication of Malaria as an Endemic Disease in the United States. *Ann Intern Med.* 1958; 48(2):428-438.

Humphreys M. *Malaria: Poverty, Race, and Public Health in the United States.* Baltimore, MD: Johns Hopkins University Press, 2001.

Stepan NL. *Eradication: Ridding the World of Diseases Forever?* Ithaca, NY: Cornell University Press; 2011. p.154.

Sledge D, Mohler G. Eliminating malaria in the American South: an analysis of the decline of malaria in 1930s Alabama. *Am J Public Health.* 2013; 103(8): 1381-1392.

Wikipedia. National Malaria Eradication Program. Wikipedia.org website. 21-Mar-2020. (Accessed 13-Jul-2021).

DDT

Carson R. *Silent Spring*. Anniversary edition. New York: Mariner Books, Houghton Mifflin Company; 2002. [Original publication date 1962].

Conis L. Beyond Silent Spring: An Alternate History of DDT. Science History. org website. 14-Feb-2017. (Accessed 10-Sep-2019).

Smallpox Eradication

Centers for Disease Control and Prevention. History of Smallpox. CDC.gov website. 30-Aug-2016. (Accessed 26-Aug-2019).

Henderson DA. Eradication: Lessons From the Past. *MMWR Morb Mortal Wkly Rep.* 1999; 48(SU01):16-22.

Bhattacharya S. Reflections on the eradication of smallpox. Lancet.com website. 8-May-2010. doi.org/10.1016/S0140-6736(10)60692-7 (Accessed 31-Aug-2019).

Stepan NL. *Eradication: Ridding the World of Diseases Forever?* Ithaca, NY: Cornell University Press; 2011. p.194-220.

Henderson DA. "A history of eradication – successes, failures, and controversies." *Lancet.* 2012; 379(9819):884-885.

Greenough P. Intimidation, Coercion and Resistance in the Final Stages of the South Asian Smallpox Eradication Campaign, 1973-1975. *Soc Sci Med.* 1995; 41(5):633-645.

Guillemin J. Smallpox: The long goodbye. The Bulletin of Atomic Scientists.org website. 21-Jul-2014. (Accessed 5-Oct-2019).

Noyce RS, Lederman S, Evans DH. Construction of an infectious horsepox virus vaccine from chemically synthesized DNA fragments. *PLoS One.* 2018; 13(1):e0188453.

Kupferschmidt K. A paper showing how to make a smallpox cousin just got published. Critics wonder why. Science Magazine.org website. 19-Jan2018. (Accessed 28-Aug-2019).

Noyce RS, Evans DH. Synthetic horsepox viruses and the continuing debate about dual use research. *PLoS Pathog.* 2018; 14(10):e1007025.

Polio Eradication

World Health Organization. Polio Endgame Strategy, 2019-2023. Eradication, Integration, Certification, and Containment. Polio Eradication.org website. 2019. (Accessed 17-Sep-2019).

World Health Organization. Polio Eradication: Report by the Director-General. Polio Eradication.org website. 8-Apr-2019. (Accessed 17-Sep-2019).

Aghamohammadi A, Abolhassani H, Kutukculer N, Wassilak SG, Pallansch MA, Kluglein S, et al. Patients with Primary Immundeficiencies Are a Reservoir of Poliovirus and a Risk to Polio Eradication. *Front Immunol.* 2017; 8:685.

Moffett DB, Llewellyn A, Singh H, Saxentoff E, Partridge J, Iakovenko M, et al. Progress Toward Poliovirus Containment Implementation – Worldwide, 2018-2019. *MMWR Morb Mortal Wkly Rep.* 2019; 68(38):825-829.

McNeil DG. "Two Strains of Polio Are Gone, but the End of the Disease Is Still Far Off." *New York Times.* 23-Oct-2019. (Accessed 24-Oct-2019).

Roberts L. "Global polio eradication falters in the final stretch." *Science.* 2020; 367(6473):14-15.

Global Polio Eradication Initiative. Global Overview – Status of Polio Eradication. 2021 Annual Session of the UNICEF Executive Board, 1-4-Jun-2021. UNICEF.org website. [No date]. (Accessed 1-Oct-2021).

Dattani S, Spooner F, Ochmann S, Roser M. Polio. Our World In Data.org website. [No date]. (Accessed 10-Jun-2023).

Chumakov K, Brechot C, Gallo RC, Plotkin S. Choosing the Right Path toward Polio Eradication. *N Engl J Med.* 2023; 388:577-579.

Bigouette JP, Henderson E, Traoré MA, Wassilak SGF, Jorba J, Mahoney F, et al. Update on Vaccine-Derived Poliovirus Outbreaks – Worldwide, January 2021-December 2022. *MMWR Morb Mortal Wkly Rep.* 2023; 72:366-371.

Lee SE, Greene SA, Burns CC, Tallis G, Wassilak SG, Bolu O. Progress Toward Poliomyelitis Eradication – Worldwide, January 2021-March 2023. *MMWR Morb Mortal Wkly Rep.* 2023; 72:517-522.

2022-2024 CDC Budgets

Centers for Disease Control and Prevention. FY 2024 Congressional Justification. CDC.gov website. 13-Mar-2023. (Accessed 5-Jun-2023).

Global Burden of Other Diseases

The Borgen Project. Top 10 Causes of Death in Developing Countries. Borgen Project.org website. 31-Mar-2018. (Accessed 17-Sep-2019).

HIV.gov. Global Statistics. HIV.gov website. 3-Aug-2022. (Accessed 27-Jun-2023).

Domestic Burden of Other Diseases

[STDs] Centers for Disease Control and Prevention. Press Release: "Reported STDs Reach All-time High for 6th Consecutive Year." CDC.gov website. 13-Apr-2021. (Accessed 27-Jun-2023).

[TB] Centers for Disease Control and Prevention. TB in the United States, 2021. CDC.gov website. 23-Mar-2023. (Accessed 23-Jun-2023).

[Foodborne Illness] Centers for Disease Control and Prevention. Burden of Foodborne Illnesses in the United States. CDC.gov website. 5-Nov-2018. (Accessed 9-Oct-2019).

[Diabetes] National Center for Health Statistics. Leading Causes of Death. CDC.gov website. 18-Jan-2023. (Accessed 27-Jun-2023).

[Cardiovascular Disease] Centers for Disease Control and Prevention. Heart Disease in the United States. CDC.gov website. 15-May-2023. (Accessed 27-Jun-2023).

CDC's Proposed Principles of Disease Elimination and Eradication
Dowdle WR. The Principles of Disease Elimination and Eradication. *MMWR Morb Mortal Wkly Rep*. 1999; 48(SU01):23-27.

Potential Conflicts Between Disease Eradication and Health Systems Development
Melgaard B, Creese A, Aylward B, Olive J-M, Maher C, Okwo-Bele J-M, et al. Disease Eradication and Health Systems Development. *MMWR Morb Mortal Wkly Rep*. 1999; 48(SU01):28-35.

Measles Resurgence in New York City and Other Urban Areas Followed by Elimination
Hutchins SS, Gindler JS, Atkinson WL, Mihalek E, Ewert E, LeBaron CW, et al. Preschool Children at High Risk for Measles: Opportunities to Vaccinate. *Am J Public Health*. 1993; 83:862-867.

LeBaron CW, Birkhead GS, Parsons P, Grabau JC, Barr-Gale L, Fuhrman J, et al. Measles Vaccination Levels of Children Enrolled in WIC during the 1991 Measles Epidemic in New York City. *Am J Public Health*. 1996; 86:1551-1556.

Birkhead GS, LeBaron CW, Parsons P, Grabau JC, Barr-Gale L, Fuhrman J, et al. The Immunization of Children Enrolled in the Special Supplemental Food Program for Women, Infants, and Children (WIC). The Impact of Different Strategies. *J Am Med Assoc*. 1995; 274(4):312-316.

Hoekstra EJ, LeBaron CW, Megaloeconomou Y, Guerro H, Byers C, Johnson-Partlow T, et al. Impact of a Large-Scale Immunization Initiative in the Special Supplemental Nutrition Program for Women, Infants, and Children (WIC). *J Am Med Assoc*. 1998; 280:1143-1147.

Orenstein WA, Papania MJ, Wharton ME. Measles Elimination in the United States. *J Infect Dis*. 2004; 189(Suppl 1):S1-3.

Guinea Worm Eradication Program
Centers for Disease Control and Prevention. Guinea Worm Eradication Program. CDC.gov website. 13-Jun-2023. (Accessed 27-Jun-2023).

Chapter Eight – Weaponizing Weakness

CDC Opioid Guideline – 2016 version

Dowell D, Haegerich TM, Chou R. CDC Guideline for Prescribing Opioids for Chronic Pain – United States, 2016. *MMWR Recomm Rep.* 2016; 65(No. RR-1):1-49.

CDC's Limited Powers

Centers for Disease Control and Prevention. The CDC Field Epidemiology Manual – Legal Considerations. CDC.gov website. 13-Dec-2018. (Accessed 16-Aug-2019).

Nicks D. "The CDC Has Less Power Than You Think, and Likes it That Way." Time Magazine.com website. 17-Oct-2014. (Accessed 30-Aug-2019).

CDC Director, CDC Staff, and How to Present Guidelines

Mandavilli A. "The C.D.C.'s New Challenge? Grappling With Imperfect Science." *New York Times.* 17-Jan-2022. (Accessed 20-Jan-2022).

Studies of Potential Effects of Prescription Limitations

Unick GJ, Rosenblum D, Mars S, Ciccarone D. Intertwined Epidemics: National Demographic Trends in Hospitalizations for Heroin- and Opioid-Related Overdoses, 1993-2009. *PLoS One.* 2013; 8(2):e54496.

Johnson H, Paulozzi L, Porucznik C, Mack K, Herter B. Decline in Drug Overdose Deaths After State Policy Changes – Florida, 2010-2012. *MMWR Morb Mortal Wkly Rep.* 2014; 63(26):569-573.

Haegerich TM, Paulozzi LJ, Manns BJ, Jones CM. What we know, and don't know, about the impact of state policy and systems-level interventions on prescription drug overdose. *Drug Alcohol Depend.* 2014; 145:34-47.

Dowell D, Zhang K, Noonan RK, Hockenberry JM. Mandatory Provider Review And Pain Clinic Laws Reduce The Amounts of Opioids Prescribed And Overdose Death Rates. *Health Aff (Millwood).* 2016; 35(10):1876-1883.

Formal System for Grading Quality of Evidence ("GRADE")

Berkman ND, Lohr KN, Ansari MT, Balk EM, Kane R, McDonagh M, et al. Grading the strength of a body of evidence when assessing health care interventions: an EPC update. *J Clin Epidemiol.* 2015; 68(11):1312-1324.

Annual Mortality Attributable to Different Conditions in 2016

[Opioid ODs] Ahmad FB, Cisewski JA, Rossen LM, Sutton P. Provisional drug overdose death counts. National Center for Health Statistics, 2023. CDC.gov website. 14-Feb-2024. (Accessed 10-Mar-2024).

[Cancer] American Cancer Society. Cancer Facts & Figures 2020. Cancer.org website. 2020. (Accessed 13-Jul-2021).

[Cardiovascular Disease] Centers for Disease Control and Prevention. Heart Disease – Heart Disease in the United States. CDC.gov website. 15-May-2023. (Accessed 28-May-2023).

CDC Director's Article Advocating for 2016 Opioid Guideline
Frieden TR, Houry D. Reducing the Risks of Relief – The CDC Opioid Prescribing Guideline. *N Engl J Med.* 2016; 374:1501-1504.

CDC Media Materials for Launch of 2016 Opioid Prescription Guideline
Centers for Disease Control and Prevention. Press Release: "CDC Releases Guideline for Prescribing Opioids for Chronic Pain – Recommendations to improve patient care, safety, and help prevent opioid misuse and overdose." CDC.gov website. 15-Mar-2016. https://archive.cdc.gov/#/details?q=https:// www.cdc.gov/media/releases/2016/p0315&start=0&rows=10&url=https:// www.cdc.gov/media/releases/2016/p0315-prescribing-opioids-guidelines. html (Accessed 22-Mar-2024).

Centers for Disease Control and Prevention. Transcript for CDC Telebriefing: Guideline for Prescribing Opioids for Chronic Pain. CDC.gov website. 15-Mar-2016. https://archive.cdc.gov/#/details?url=https://www.cdc.gov/ media/releases/2016/t0315-prescribing-opioids-guidelines.html (Accessed 22-Mar-2024).

Media Reports about Issuance of 2016 Opioid Prescription Guideline
Szabo L. "Doctors told to avoid prescribing opiates for chronic pain." *USA TODAY.* 16-Mar-2016. (Accessed 26-Feb-2022).

Demirjian K, Bernstein L. "CDC warns doctors about the dangers of prescribing opioid painkillers." *Washington Post.* 15-Mar-2016. (Accessed 26-Feb-2022).

Tavernise S. "C.D.C. Painkiller Guidelines Aim to Reduce Addiction Risk." *New York Times.* 15-Mar-2016. (Accessed 26-Feb-2022).

Zalkind S. "CDC issues guidelines against opioid prescriptions to treat chronic pain." *The Guardian.* 17-Mar-2016. (Accessed 26-Feb-2022).

Widespread Implementation of CDC Opioid Guideline
[State Laws]
National Conference of State Legislatures. Prescribing policies: states confront opioid overdose epidemic. NCSL.org website. 30-Jun-2019. (Accessed 26-Feb-2022).

[Congressional Bill CARA 2.0]
Shatterproof. "5 things you need to know about CARA 2.0." Shatterproof.org website. 1-Mar-2018. (Accessed 27-Aug-2019).

GovTrack. "H.R. 5311 (115th) CARA 2.0 Act of 2018." GovTrack.us website. [No date]. (Accessed 27-Aug-2019).

[Insurance]

Blue Cross Blue Shield. Press Release: "Capital BlueCross announces significant reduction in opioids dispensed following prescription limitations." BCBS. com website. 22-Mar-2018. (Accessed 27-Aug-2019).

Cigna. Press Release: "Use of prescribed opioids down nearly 12 percent over 12 months among Cigna customers." Cigna.com website. 6-Apr-2017. (Accessed 27-Aug-2019).

United Healthcare. 2019 Opioid Readiness: United Healthcare Medicare Advantage and Prescription Drug Plans – Quick Reference Guide. UHC Provider.com website. [No date]. (Accessed 27-Aug-2019).

[Medicare]

CMS Medicare Learning Network. A prescriber's guide to the new Medicare Part D opioid overutilization policies for 2019. Center for Medicare Services (CMS.gov) website. 1-Nov-2018. (Accessed 27-Aug-2019).

Hartung DM, Johnston K, Geddes J, Leichtling G, Priest KC, Korthuis PT. Buprenorphine Coverage in the Medicare Part D Program for 2007 to 2018. *J Am Med Assoc.* 2019; 321(6):607-609.

Hoffman J. "Medicare is cracking down on opioids. Doctors fear pain patients will suffer." *New York Times.* 27-Mar-2018. (Accessed 1-Oct-2019).

[Medicaid]

Ballotpedia. Opiate prescription limits and policies by state. Ballotpedia.org website. Aug-2019. (Accessed 27-Aug-2019).

Diep F. "Oregon considers ending coverage of opioid painkillers for chronic pain." *Pacific Standard.* 15-Aug-2018. (Accessed 1-Oct-2019).

[Pharmacies]

[Express Scripts] Miller K. Putting the Brakes on the Opioid Epidemic. Lehigh Valley Business Coalition on Healthcare (lvbch.com) website. 26-Oct-2017. (Accessed 27-Aug-2019).

[CVS] CVS Caremark® Opioid Quantity Limits – Pharmacy Reference Guide. Caremark.com website. 2018. (Accessed 27-Aug-2019).

[Walmart] Romo V. "Walmart will implement new opioid prescription limits by end of summer." *National Public Radio (NPR).* NPR.org website. 8-May-2018. (Accessed 1-Oct-2019).

[Veterans Administration and Department of Defense] Veterans Administration & Department of Defense. VA/DoD Clinical Practice Guideline for Opioid Therapy for Chronic Pain Version 3.0. Feb 2017 VA.gov website. Feb-2017. (Accessed 27-Aug-2019).

[White House Opioid Initiative]

White House. "Fact Sheets: President Donald J. Trump's Initiative to Stop Opioid Abuse and Reduce Drug Supply and Demand." White House.gov website. 24-Oct-2018. (Accessed 27-Aug-2019).

[Drug Enforcement Administration Letter to Human Rights Watch 14-Sep-2018]

Human Rights Watch. "Not Allowed to Be Compassionate" Chronic Pain, the Overdose Crisis, and Unintended Harms in the US. 2018. Annex I. p.88. Human Rights Watch (HRW.org) website. (Accessed 28-Aug-2019).

Reduction in Opioid Prescriptions Following Issuance of CDC Opioid Prescription Guideline

Bohnert ASB, Guy GP, Losby JL. Opioid Prescribing in the United States Before and After the Centers for Disease Control and Prevention's 2016 Opioid Guideline. *Ann Intern Med.* 2018; 169(6):367-375.

Scherrer JF, Tucker J, Salas J, Zhang Z, Grucza R. Comparison of Opioids Prescribed for Patients at Risk for Opioid Misuse Before and After Publication of the Centers for Disease Control and Prevention's Opioid Prescribing Guidelines. *JAMA Netw Open.* 2020; 3(12):e2027481.

Goldstick JE, Guy GP, Losby JL, Baldwin G, Myers M, Bohnert ASB. Changes in Initial Opioid Prescribing Practices After the 2016 Release of the CDC Guideline for Prescribing Opioids for Chronic Pain. *JAMA Netw Open.* 2021; 4(7):e2116860.

Stein BD, Taylor EA, Sheng F, Dick AW, Vaiana M, Sorbero M. Change in Per Capita Opioid Prescriptions Filled at Retail Pharmacies, 2008-2009 to 2017-2018. *Ann Intern Med.* 2022; 175(2):299-302.

CDC Collaboration with Law Enforcement Authorities on Opioids

Schuchat A, Houry D, Guy GP. New Data on Opioid Use and Prescribing in the United States. *J Am Med Assoc.* 2017; 318(5):425-426.

Concerns about Potential Effects of Rigid Opioid Prescription Controls

Kroenke K, Cheville A. Management of Chronic Pain in the Aftermath of the Opioid Backlash. *J Am Med Assoc.* 2017; 317(23):2365-2366.

Kertesz SG, Gordon AJ. A crisis of opioids and the limits of prescription control: United States. *Addiction.* 2019; 114:169-180.

Yang YT, Haffajee RL. Murder Liability for Prescribing Opioids: A Way Forward? *Mayo Clin Proc.* 2016; 91(10):1331-1335.

Young KD. Study Finds Sharp Drop in Opioid Scripts Among Most Specialists. Medscape.com website. 4-Jan-2022. (Accessed 26-Feb-2022).

Chapter Nine – A Comedy of Errors, or Cruel and Inhuman Punishment?

Examples of Other CDC Clinical Guidelines

[Tuberculosis] Nahid P, Dorman SE, Alipanah N, Barry PM, Brozek JL, Cattamanchi A, et al. Official American Thoracic Society/Centers for Disease Control and Prevention/Infectious Disease Society of America Clinical Practice Guidelines: Treatment of Drug-Susceptible Tuberculosis. *Clin Infect Dis.* 2016; 63(7):e147-e195.

[HIV] HIVInfo. Clinical Guidelines. HIVInfo.nih.gov website. [No date]. (Accessed 28-Jun-2023).

[Immunization] Centers for Disease Control and Prevention. Advisory Committee on Immunization Practices. CDC.gov website. 19-May-2023. (Accessed 28-Jun-2023).

Initial Reactions to CDC Opioid Guideline

American Medical Association. What physicians are saying about the new CDC opioid guidelines. American Medical Association (ama-assnb.org) website. 16-Mar-2016. (Accessed 27-Aug-2019).

Renthal W. Seeking Balance Between Pain Relief and Safety – CDC Issues New Opioid-Prescribing Guidelines. *JAMA Neurol.* 2016; 73(5):513-514.

Anecdotes of Problems with Opioid Dose Limitation or Discontinuation

Webster LR. President's Message – Pain and suicide: the other side of the opioid story. *Pain Med.* 2014; 15(3):345-346.

Weeks WB. Hailey – my little sister was 49 when she died. *J Am Med Assoc.* 2016; 316(19):1975-1976.

Glod SA. The other victims of the opioid epidemic. *N Engl J Med.* 2017; 22:2101-2102.

Llorente E. "As doctors taper or end opioid prescriptions, many patients driven to despair, suicide." Fox News.com website. 10-Dec-2018. (Accessed 9-Oct-2019).

Rubin R. Limits on opioid prescribing leave patients with chronic pain vulnerable. *J Am Med Assoc.* 2019; 321(21):2059-2062.

Redmon J. "Georgia pain doctor stays busy amid opioid abuse epidemic. Increased risks, scrutiny weigh heavily on Augusta physician." *Atlanta Journal Constitution.* 1-Dec-2019. (Accessed 26-Dec-2019).

Risk of Suicide from Opioid Reduction/Discontinuation

Demidenko MI, Dobscha SK, Morasco BJ, Meath THA, Ilgen MA, Lovejoy TI. Suicidal ideation and suicidal self-directed violence following clinician-initiated prescription opioid discontinuation among long-term opioid users. *Gen Hosp Psychiatry*. 2017; 47:29-35.

Oliva EM, Bowe T, Manhapra A, Kertesz S, Hah JM, Henderson P, et al. Associations between stopping prescriptions for opioids, length of opioid treatment, and overdose or suicide deaths in US veterans: observational evaluation. *BMJ*. 2020; 368:m283.

Hallvik SE, El Ibrahimi S, Johnston K, Geddes J, Leichtling G, Korthuis PT, et al. Patient outcomes after opioid dose reduction among patients with chronic opioid therapy. *Pain*. 2022; 163(1):83-90.

Limitations of Opioid Access for Cancer Patients

American Cancer Society Cancer Action Network and Patient Quality of Life Coalition. Key Findings Summary: Opioid Access Research Project. Fight Cancer.org website. [No date]. (Accessed 8-Aug-2020).

Page R, Blanchard E. Opioids and Cancer Pain: Patients' Needs and Access Challenges. *J Oncol Pract*. 2019; 15(5):229-231.

Vitzthum LK, Riviere P, Murphy JD. Managing Cancer Pain During the Opioid Epidemic – Balancing Caution and Compassion. *JAMA Oncol*. 2020; 6(7):1103-1104.

Chino F, Kamal A, Chino J. Incidence of Opioid-Associated Deaths in Cancer Survivors in the United States, 2006-2016: A Population Study of the Opioid Epidemic. *JAMA Oncol*. 2020; 6(7):1100-1102.

Chen Y, Spillane S, Shiels MS, Young L, Quach D, Berrington de González A, et al. Trends in Opioid Use Among Cancer Patients in the United States: 2013-2018. *JNCI Cancer Spectr*. 2022; 6(1):pkab095.

Online Survey of Pain Patients

Pain News Network. 2017 CDC Survey Results. Pain News Network.org website. [No date]. (Accessed 28-Feb-2022).

Limitation of Opioid Access for Chronic Pain Patients

American Board of Pain Medicine. Second Annual Survey of Pain Medicine Specialists Highlights Continued Plight of Patients with Pain, and Barriers to Providing Multidiscplinary, Non-Opioid Care. American Board of Pain Medicine (ABPM.org) website. [No date]. (Accessed 8-Aug-2020).

Estimated Number of Persons with Chronic Pain

Rikard SM, Strahan AE, Schmit KM, Guy GP Jr. Chronic Pain Among Adults – United States, 2019-2021. *MMWR Morb Mortal Wkly Rep.* 2023; 72:379-385.

Advocacy Group for Those with Chronic Pain

Don't Punish Pain Rally. Don't Punish Pain Rally.com website. [No date]. (Accessed 26-Aug-2019).

Marill MC. "The unseen victims of the opioid crisis are starting to rebel." Wired.com website. 21-May-2019. (Accessed 27-Aug-2019).

Professional/Organizational Criticism of CDC Opioid Guideline & Related News Reports

Watson J. Abandoned to Pain: Has Opioid Access Become Too Restrictive? Medscape.com website. 28-Sep-2018. (Accessed 1-Oct-2019).

Lampner C. The Unintended Consequences of the CDC Opioid Guideline According to Pain Management Specialists. Clinical Pain Advisor.com website. 30-Oct-2018. (Accessed 27-Aug-2019).

Anson P. AMA: 'Inappropriate Use' of CDC Guideline Should Stop. *Pain News Network.* 14-Nov-2018. (Accessed 27-Aug-2019).

O'Reilly KB. How the CDC's opioid prescribing guidance went astray. American Medical Association (ama-assn.org) website. 26-Apr-2019. (Accessed 28-Jun-2023).

Kroenke K, Alford DP, Argoff C, Canlas B, Covington E, Frank JW, et al. Challenges with implementing the Centers for Disease Control and Prevention Opioid Guideline: A Consensus Panel Report. *Pain Med.* 2019; 20(4):724-735.

U.S. Department of Health and Human Services. Pain Management Best Practices Inter-Agency Task Force Report: Updates, Gaps, Inconsistencies, and Recommendations. HHS.gov website. 9-May-2019. (Accessed 27-Aug-2019).

Health Professionals for Patients in Pain (HP3). Letter to CDC Director: "Health Professionals Call on the CDC to Address Misapplication of its Guideline on Opioids for Chronic Pain through Public Clarification and Impact Evaluation." HP3.org website. 6-Mar-2019. (Accessed 27-Aug-2019).

Hoffman J, Goodnough A. "Good News: Opioid Prescribing Fell. The Bad? Pain Patients Suffer, Doctors Say. Doctors and insurers are using federal guidelines as cover to turn away patients, experts tell the C.D.C. and Congress." *New York Times.* 6-Mar-2019. (Accessed 27-Aug-2019).

Bernstein L. "Health-care providers say CDC's opioid guidelines are harming pain patients." *Washington Post.* 6-Mar-2019. (Accessed 27-Aug-2019).

Scientific Critiques of CDC Opioid Guideline

Busse JW, Juulink D, Guyatt GH. Addressing the limitations of the CDC guideline for prescribing opioids for chronic noncancer pain. *CMAJ*. 2016; 188(17-18):1210-1211.

Schatman ME, Ziegler SJ. Pain management, prescription opioid mortality, and the CDC: is the devil in the data? *J Pain Res*. 2017; 10:2489-2495.

Jay GW, Barkin RL. Perspectives on the opioid crisis from pain medicine clinicians. *Dis Mon*. 2018; 64(10):451-466.

Trends in Opioid Prescription Counts Compared with Overdose Death Rates

Centers for Disease Control and Prevention. Changes in Opioid Prescribing Practices. CDC.gov website. 13-Aug-2019. (Accessed 28-Aug-2019).

National Institute of Drug Abuse. Overdose Death Rates. Drug Abuse.gov website. 9-Feb-2023. (Accessed 28-Jun-2023).

Massachusetts Department of Health. An Assessment of Opioid-Related Deaths in Massachusetts (2013-2014). Mass.gov website. 15-Sep-2016. (Accessed 28-Aug-2019).

Centers for Disease Control and Prevention. 2018 Annual Surveillance Report of Drug-Related Risks and Outcomes – United States. Surveillance Special Report. Centers for Disease Control and Prevention, U.S. Department of Health and Human Services. CDC.gov website. 31-Aug-2018. (Accessed 26-Aug-2019).

Schieber LZ, Guy GP, Seth P, Young R, Mattson CL, Mikosz CA, Schieber RA. Trends and Patterns of Geographic Variation in Opioid Prescribing Practices by State, United States, 2006-2017. *JAMA Netw Open*. 2019; 2(3):e190665.

Strickler GK, Kreiner PW, Halpin JF, Doyle E, Paulozzi LJ. Opioid Prescribing Behaviors – Prescription Behavior Surveillance System, 11 States, 2010-2016. *MMWR Morb Mortal Surveill Summ*. 2020; 69(No. SS-1):1-14.

Characteristics of Persons Prescribed Opioids Compared with Those Who Overdose on Opioids

Centers for Disease Control and Prevention. 2018 Annual Surveillance Report of Drug-Related Risks and Outcomes – United States. Surveillance Special Report. Centers for Disease Control and Prevention, U.S. Department of Health and Human Services. CDC.gov website. 31-Aug-2018. (Accessed 28-Aug-2019).

Kaiser Family Foundation. Opioid Overdose Deaths. Kaiser Family Foundation (KFF.org) website. 2017. (Accessed 28-Aug-2019).

Gomes T, Tadrous M, Mamdani MM, Paterson JM, Juulink DN. The Burden of Opioid-Related Mortality in the United States. *JAMA Netw Open.* 2018; 1(2):e180217.

Rigg KK, Monnat SM. Comparing Characteristics of Prescription Painkiller Misusers and Heroin Users in the United States. *Addict Behav.* 2015; 51:106-112.

Opioid Prescription Limitations, Decreased Access, and Increased Illicit Opioid Use

Unick GJ, Rosenblum D, Mars S, Ciccarone D. Intertwined Epidemics: National Demographic Trends in Hospitalizations for Heroin- and Opioid-Related Overdoses, 1993-2009. *PLoS One.* 2013; 8(2):e54496.

Ebbert JO, Philpot LM, Clements CM, Lovely JK, Nicholson WT, Jenkins SM, et al. Attitudes, Beliefs, Practices, and Concerns Among Clinicians Prescribing Opioids in a Large Academic Institution. *Pain Med.* 2018; 19(9):1790-1798.

Cicero TJ, Ellis MS, Kasper ZA. Increased use of heroin as an initiating opioid of abuse. *Addict Behav.* 2017; 74:63-66.

Cicero TJ, Kasper ZA, Ellis MS. Increased use of heroin as an initiating opioid of abuse: further considerations and policy considerations. *Addict Behav.* 2018; 87:267-271.

Martin J, Cunliffe J, Décary-Hétu D, Aldridge J. Effect of restricting the legal supply of prescription opioids on buying through online illicit market-places: interrupted time series analysis. *BMJ.* 2018; 361:k2270.

Mark TL, Parish W. Opioid medication discontinuation and risk of adverse opioid-related health events. *J Subst Abuse Treat.* 2019; 103:58-63.

Lagisetty PA, Healy N, Garpestal C, Jannausch M, Tipirneni R, Bohnert ASB. Access to Primary Care Clinics for Patients With Chronic Pain Receiving Opioids. *JAMA Netw Open.* 2019; 2(7):e196928.

McGinty EE, Stone EM, Kennedy-Hendricks A, Bachhuber MA, Barry CL. Medication for Opioid Use Disorder: A National Survey of Primary Care Physicians. *Ann Intern Med.* 2020; 173(2):160-162.

Coffin PO, Rowe C, Oman N, Sinchek K, Santos G-M, Faul M, et al. Illicit opioid use following changes in opioids prescribed for chronic non-cancer pain. *PLoS One.* 2020; 15(5):e0232538.

Lagisetty P, Macleod C, Thomas J, Slat S, Kehne A, Heisler M, et al. Assessing reasons for decreased primary care access for individuals on prescribed opioids: an audit study. *Pain.* 2021; 162(5):1379-1386.

FDA Warning Against Sudden Discontinuation of Opioid Pain Medicines
Food and Drug Administation. FDA identifies harm reported from sudden
discontinuation of opioid pain medicines and requires label changes to
guide prescribers on gradual, individualized tapering – FDA Drug Safety
Communication. FDA.gov website. 9-Apr-2019. (Accessed 10-Mar-2022).

Lack of Opioid Treatment Access and Increased Adverse Events/Mortality
Jones CW, Christman Z, Smith CM, Safferman MR, Salzman M, Baston K, et
al. Comparison between buprenorphine provider availability and opioid
deaths among US counties. *J Subst Abuse Treat.* 2018; 93:19-25.
Haffajee R, Lin LA, Bohnert ASB, Goldstick JE. Characteristics of US
Counties With High Opioid Overdose Mortality and Low Capacity to
Deliver Medications for Opioid Use Disorder. *JAMA Netw Open.* 2019;
2(6):e196373.
Langabeer JR, Gourishankar A, Chambers KA, Giri S, Madu R, Champagne-
Langabeer T. Disparities between US opioid overdose deaths and treatment capacity: a geospatial and descriptive analysis. *J Addict Med.* 2019;
13(6):476-482.
Gordon KS, Manhapra A, Crystal S, Dziura J, Edelman EJ, Skanderson M, et
al. All-cause mortality among males living with and without HIV initiating
long-term opioid therapy, and its association with opioid dose, opioid
interruption and other factors. *Drug Alcohol Depend.* 2020; 216:108291.
Oliva EM, Bowe T, Manhapra A, Kertesz S, Hah JM, Henderson P, et al.
Associations between stopping prescriptions for opioids, length of opioid
treatment, and overdose or suicide deaths in US veterans: observational
evaluation. *BMJ.* 2020; 368:m283.
Agnoli A, Xing G, Tancredi DJ, Magnan E, Jerant A, Fenton JJ. Association of
Dose Tapering With Overdose or Mental Health Crisis Among Patients
Prescribed Long-term Opioids. *J Am Med Assoc.* 2021; 326(5):411-419.

**Modeling Studies of Impact of Prescription Drug Controls on Addiction/
Overdose Rates**
Pitt AL, Humphrey K, Brandeau ML. Modeling health benefits and harms of
public policy responses to the US opioid epidemic. *Am J Public Health.*
2018; 108(10):1394-1400.
Chen Q, Larochelle MR, Weaver DT, Lietz AP, Mueller PP, Mercaldo S, et al.
Prevention of prescription opioid misuse and projected overdose deaths in
the United States. *JAMA Netw Open.* 2019; 2(2):e187621.

Human Rights Watch Report

Human Rights Watch. "Not Allowed to Be Compassionate" Chronic Pain, the Overdose Crisis, and Unintended Harms in the US. Human Rights Watch (HRW.org) website. 2018. (Accessed 28-Aug-2019).

Chapter Ten – The Power of Persuasion

Letters of Clarification of Guideline

Letter of clarification of CDC Opioid Guideline concerning cancer survivors and persons with sickle cell disease. 28-Feb-2019. American Society of Clinical Oncology (ASCO.org) website. https://www.asco.org/sites/new-www.asco.org/files/content-files/advocacy-and-policy/documents/2019-CDC-Opioid-Guideline-Clarification-Letter-to-ASCO-ASH-NCCN.pdf (Accessed 22-Mar-2024).

CDC Director's letter to Health Professionals for Patients in Pain.10-Apr-2019. https://img1.wsimg.com/blobby/go/3d70257f-a143-4a5b-b9df-7d265df0d3d/downloads/Alford%20Final%20.pdf?ver=1556148791199 (Accessed 22-Mar-2024).

HHS Guide for Clinicians on Opioid Reduction/Discontinuance

U.S. Department of Health and Human Services. HHS guide for clinicians on the appropriate dosage reduction or discontinuation of long-term opioid analgesics. National Institute on Drug Abuse/National Institute of Health (NIDA.NIH.gov) website. Oct-2019. (Accessed 28-Jun-2023).

Dowell D, Compton WM, Giroir BP. Patient-Centered Reduction or Discontinuation of Long-Term Opioid Analgesics. *J Am Med Assoc*. 2019; 322(19):1855-1856.

Goodnough A. "Health Officials Urge Caution in Reducing Opioids of Pain Patients." *New York Times*. 10-Oct-2019. (Accessed 13-Jul-2021).

Frank JW, Lovejoy TI, Becker WC, Morasco BJ, Koenig CJ, Hoffecker L, et al. Patient Outcomes in Dose Reduction or Discontinuation of Long-Term Opioid Therapy: A Systematic Review. *Ann Intern Med*. 2017; 167:181-191.

CDC Guideline Authors' Article/Interview in *New England Journal of Medicine*

Dowell D, Taegerich T, Chou R. Perspective: No Shortcut to Safer Opioid Prescribing. *N Engl J Med*. 2019; 380:2285-2287.

2018 Overdose Death Numbers

Ahmad FB, Cisewski JA, Rossen LM, Sutton P. Provisional drug overdose death counts. National Center for Health Statistics, 2024. CDC.gov website. 14-Feb-2024. (Accessed 10-Mar-2024).

Goodnough A, Katz J, Sanger-Katz M. "Drug Overdose Deaths Drop in U.S. for First Time Since 1990." *New York Times.* 17-Jul-2019. (Accessed 24-Aug-2019).

Hedegaard H, Miniño AM, Warner M. Drug overdose deaths in the United States, 1999–2018. NCHS Data Brief, no 356. Hyattsville, MD: National Center for Health Statistics. 2020. CDC.gov website. (Accessed 8-Aug-2020).

Wilson N, Kariisa M, Seth P, Smith H IV, Davis NL. Drug and Opioid-Involved Overdose Deaths – United States, 2017-2018. *MMWR Morb Mortal Wkly Rep.* 2020; 69:290-297.

Graph of Opioid-Related Overdose Deaths

National Institute on Drug Abuse. Overdose Death Rates: Drug Overdoses Data Document. Drug Abuse.gov website. 9-Feb-2023. (Accessed 27-Jun-2023).

Ahmad FB, Cisewski JA, Rossen LM, Sutton P. Provisional drug overdose death counts. National Center for Health Statistics, 2023. CDC.gov website. 14-Feb-2024. (Accessed 10-Mar-2024).

National Center for Health Statistics. Provisional Data Shows U.S. Drug Overdose Deaths Top 100,000 in 2022. CDC.gov website. 18-May-2023. (Accessed 5-Jun-2023).

Dowell D, Haegerich TM, Chou R. CDC Guideline for Prescribing Opioids for Chronic Pain – United States, 2016. *MMWR Recomm Rep.* 2016; 65 (No. RR-1):1-49.

Chapter Eleven – Bending the Curve

Issues in Evaluating Overdose Death Rates

Warner M, Paulozzi LJ, Nolte KB, Davis GG, Nelson LS. State variation in certifying manner of death and drugs involved in drug intoxication deaths. *Acta Forensic Pathol.* 2013; 3(2):231-237.

Stone DM, Holland KM, Bartholow B, Logan JE, McIntosh WLW, Trudeau A, et al. Deciphering Suicide and Other Manners of Death Associated with Drug Intoxication: A Centers for Disease Control and Prevention Consultation Meeting Summary. *Am J Public Health.* 2017; 107(8):1233-1239.

Schatman ME, Ziegler SJ. Pain management, prescription opioid mortality, and the CDC: is the devil in the data? *J Pain Res.* 2017; 10:2489-2495.

Hannah HA, Arambula K, Ereman R, Harris D, Torres A, Willis M. Using local toxicology data for drug overdose mortality surveillance. *Online J Public Health Inform.* 2017; 9(1):e143.

Human Rights Watch. "Poor Data: An Impediment to an Effective Response to the Opioid Crisis" p.71-77 in "Not Allowed to Be Compassionate" Chronic Pain, the Overdose Crisis, and Unintended Harms in the US. 2018. Human Rights Watch (HRW.org) website. (Accessed 28-Aug-2019).

Ahmad FB, Cisewski JA, Rossen LM, Sutton P. Provisional drug overdose death counts. National Center for Health Statistics, 2023. CDC.gov website. 14-Feb-2024. (Accessed 10-Mar-2024).

Rossen LM, Ahmad FB, Spencer MR, Warner M, Sutton P. Methods to Adjust Provisional Counts of Drug Overdose Deaths for Underreporting. Vital Statistics Rapid Release; no 6. Hyattsville, MD. National Center for Health Statistics. CDC.gov website. August 2018. (Accessed 13-Jul-2021).

Hedegaard H, Bastian BA, Trinidad JP, Warner M. Drugs most frequently involved in drug overdose deaths: United States, 2011-2016. National Vital Statistics Reports; vol 67 no 9. Hyattsville, MD: National Center for Health Statistics. CDC.gov website. 2018. (Accessed 22-March-2024).

Gladden RM, O'Donnell J, Mattson CL, Seth P. Changes in Opioid-Involved Overdose Deaths by Opioid Type and Presence of Benzodiazepines, Cocaine, and Methamphetamine – 25 States, July-December 2017 to January-June 2018. *MMWR Morb Mortal Wkly Rep.* 2019; 68(34):737-744.

Anecdotes of Multidrug Overdoses

Barron J. "Medical Examiner Rules Heath Ledger's Death Accidental." *New York Times.* 7-Feb-2008. (Accessed 28-Jun-2023).

Wikipedia. Philip Seymour Hoffman. Wikipedia.org website. 5-Jul-2021. (Accessed 13-Jul-2021).

2019 & 2020 Overdose Death Rates

Katz J, Goodnough A, Sanger-Katz M. "In the Shadow of Pandemic, U.S. Drug Overdose Deaths Resurge to Record." *New York Times.* 15-July-2020. (Accessed 13-Jul-2021).

National Institute on Drug Abuse. Overdose Death Rates: Drug Overdoses Data Document. Drug Abuse.gov website. 9-Feb-2023. (Accessed 27-Jun-2023).

Haley DF, Saitz R. The Opioid Epidemic During the COVID-19 Pandemic. *J Am Med Assoc.* 2020; 324(16):1615-1617.

Wainright JJ, Mikre M, Whitley P, Dawson E, Huskey A, Lukowiak A, et al. Analysis of Drug Test Results Before and After the US Declaration of a National Emergency Concerning the COVID-19 Outbreak. *J Am Med Assoc.* 2020; 324(16):1674-1677.

Ochalek TA, Cumpston KL, Wills BK, Gal TS, Moeller FG. Nonfatal Opioid Overdoses at an Urban Emergency Department During the COVID-19 Pandemic. *J Am Med Assoc.* 2020; 324(16):1673-1674.

Stephenson J. Drug Overdose Deaths Head Toward Record Number in 2020, CDC Warns. *JAMA Health Forum.* 2020;1(10):e201318.

Friedman J, Beletsky L, Schriger DL. Overdose-Related Cardiac Arrests Observed by Emergency Medical Services During the US COVID-19 Epidemic. *JAMA Psychiatry.* 2021; 78(5):562-564.

Hedgaard H, Miniño AM, Warner M. Drug overdose deaths in the United States, 1999-2019. NCHS Data Brief. no 394. Hyattsville, MD: National Center for Health Statistics. 2020. CDC.gov website. 22-Dec-2020. (Accessed 13-Jul-2021).

Mattson CL, Tanz LJ, Quinn K, Kariisa M, Patel P, Davis NL. Trends and Geographic Patterns in Drug and Synthetic Opioid Overdose Deaths – United States, 2013-2019. *MMWR Morb Mortal Wkly Rep.* 2021; 70:202-207.

Ahmad FB, Cisewski JA, Rossen LM, Sutton P. Provisional drug overdose death counts. National Center for Health Statistics, 2023. CDC.gov website. 14-Feb-2024. (Accessed 10-Mar-2024).

Katz J, Sanger-Katz M. "Drug Deaths Spiked by 30 Percent Last Year, Surpassing 90,000." *New York Times.* 14-Jul-2021. (Accessed 14-Jul-2021).

Chappell B. "Drug Overdoses Killed A Record Number Of Americans In 2020, Jumping By Nearly 30%." *National Public Radio (NPR).* National Public Radio (NPR.org) website. 14-Jul-2021. (Accessed 15-Jul-2021).

Kariisa M, Davis NL, Kumar S, Seth P, Mattson CL Chowdhury F, et al. Vital Signs: Drug Overdose Deaths, by Selected Sociodemographic and Social Determinants of Health Characteristics – 25 States and the District of Columbia, 2019-2020. *MMWR Morb Mortal Wkly Rep.* 2022; 71(29):940-947.

Bruzelius E, Martins SS. US Trends in Drug Overdose Mortality Among Pregnant and Postpartum Persons, 2017-2020. *J Am Med Assoc.* 2022; 328(21):2159-2161.

Social/Racial/Ethnic Patterns in 2019-2020 Opioid Overdoses

Friedman J, Mann NC, Hansen H, Bourgois P, Braslow J, Bui AAT, et al. Racial/Ethnic, Social, and Geographic Trends in Overdose-Associated Cardiac Arrests Observed by US Emergency Medical Services During the COVID-19 Pandemic. *JAMA Psychiatry.* 2021; 78(8):886-895.

Opioid Deaths Compared with Covid Deaths in a Major City

Baker M. "Overdoses Have Killed More Than Three Times as Many People as COVID-19 in San Francisco." *San Francisco Public Press.* 17-Dec-2020. (Accessed 13-Jul-2021).

Fuller T. "San Francisco Contends With a Different Sort of Epidemic: Drug Deaths." *New York Times.* 23-Apr-2021. (Accessed 17-Jun-2021).

The "Drug Bust Paradox"

Acharya JC, Lyons BC, Murthy V, Stanley J, Babcock C, Jackson K, et al. An Emergency Preparedness Response to Opioid-Prescribing Enforcement Actions in Maryland, 2018-2019. *Public Health Rep.* 2021; 136(1_suppl):9S-17S.

Ray B, Korzeniewski SJ, Mohler G, Carroll JJ, Del Pozo B, Victor G, et al. Spatiotemporal Analysis Exploring the Effect of Law Enforcement Drug Market Disruptions on Overdose, Indianapolis, Indiana, 2020-2021. *Am J Public Health.* 2023; 113:750-758.

Dasgupta N. We Can't Arrest Our Way Out of Overdose: The Drug Bust Paradox. *Am J Public Health.* 2023; 113:708.

Facher L. "'The drug bust paradox': Study shows opioid deaths double after police action." *STAT.* Statnews.com website. 13-Jun-2023. (Accessed 26-Jun-2023).

CDC Health Alert Network Notification about 2019-2020 Opioid Epidemic

Centers for Disease Control and Prevention. Health Advisory: Increase in Fatal Drug Overdoses Across the United States Driven by Synthetic Opioids Before and After the COVID-19 Pandemic. CDCHAN-00438. Emergency.cdc.gov website. 17-Dec-2020. (Accessed 17-Jun-2021).

Naloxone Distribution Impact on Opioid Overdose Deaths and Hospitalizations Rates

Walley AY, Xuan Z, Hackman HH, Quinn E, Doe-Simkins M, Sorensen-Alawad A, et al. Opioid overdose rates and implementation of overdose education and nasal naloxone distribution in Massachusetts: interrupted time series. *BMJ.* 2013; 346:F174.

McClellan C, Lambdin BH, Ali MM, Mutter R, Davis CS, Wheeler E, et al. Opioid-overdose laws association with opioid use and overdose mortality. *Addict Behav.* 2018; 86:90-95.

Collins AB, Ndoye CD, Arene-Morley D, Marshall BDL. Addressing co-occurring public health emergencies: The importance of naloxone distribution in the era of COVID-19. *Int J Drug Policy.* 2020; 83:102872.

Nonfatal Overdose as Risk Factor for Subsequent Fatal Overdose

Olfson M, Wall M, Wang S, Crystal S, Blanco C. Risks of fatal opioid overdose during the first year following nonfatal overdose. *Drug Alcohol Depend.* 2018; 190:112-119.

Krawczyk N, Eisenberg M, Schneider KE, Richards TM, Lyons BC, Jackson K, et al. Predictors of Overdose Death Among High-Risk Emergency Department Patients With Substance-Related Encounters: A Data Linkage Cohort Study. *Ann Emerg Med.* 2020; 75(1):1-12.

Gupta R, Holtgrave DR. A National Tracking System for Nonfatal Drug Overdoses. *J Am Med Assoc.* 2022; 328(3):239-240.

Naloxone Prescribing

Guy GPO, Haegerich TM, Evans ME, Losby JL, Young R, Jones CM. Vital Signs: Pharmacy-Based Naloxone Dispensing – United States, 2012-2018. *MMWR Morb Mortal Wkly Rep.* 2019; 68(31):679-686.

Ochalek TA, Cumpston KL, Wills BK, Gal TS, Moeller FG. Nonfatal Opioid Overdoses at an Urban Emergency Department During the COVID-19 Pandemic. *J Am Med Assoc.* 2020; 324(16):1673-1674.

O'Donoghue A, Biswas N, Dechen T, Anderson TS, Talmor N, Punnamaraju A, et al. Trends in Filled Naloxone Prescriptions Before and During the COVID-19 Pandemic in the United States. *JAMA Health Forum.* 2021; 2(5):e210393.

Higher-Dose Naloxone Nasal Spray (Kloxxado) for Opioid Overdose. *The Medical Letter on Drugs and Therapeutics.* 20-Sep-2021. 2021; 63(1633):151-152.

Khoury D, Preiss A, Geiger P, Anwar M, Conway KP. Increases in Naloxone Administrations by Emergency Medical Services Providers During the COVID-19 Pandemic: Retrospective Time Series Study. *JMIR Public Health Surveill.* 2021; 7(5):e29298.

Barnett ML, Meara E, Lewinson T, Hardy B, Chyn D, Onsando M, et al. Racial Inequality in Receipt of Medications for Opioid Disorder. *N Engl J Med.* 2023; 388:1779-1789.

2021 Overdose Estimates

Langmaid V. "US reaches record high of more than 96,000 drug overdose deaths in a 12-month period, CDC data show." CNN.com website. 13-Oct-2021. (Accessed 12-Nov-2021).

Rabin RC. "Overdose Deaths Reached Record High as the Pandemic Spread." *New York Times.* 17-Nov-2021. (Accessed 24-Nov-2021).

O'Donnell J, Tanz LJ, Gladden RM, Davis NL, Bitting J. Trends in and Characteristics of Drug Overdose Deaths Involving Illicitly Manufactured Fentanyls – United States, 2019-2020. *MMWR Morb Mortal Wkly Rep.* 2021; 70:1740-1746.

MacGuill D. "Did Fentanyl Overdose Become Top Cause of Death for Adults Aged 18-45 in the US?" *Snopes.* 21-Dec-2021. (Accessed 10-Mar-2022).

Commission on Combating Synthetic Opioid Trafficking. Final Report. Rand.org website. 2-Feb-2022. p.1. (Accessed 9-Feb-2022).

Ahmad FB, Cisewski JA, Rossen LM, Sutton P. Provisional drug overdose death counts. National Center for Health Statistics, 2024. CDC.gov website. 14-Feb-2024. (Accessed 10-Mar-2024).

Tanz LJ, Dinwiddie AT, Mattson CL, O'Donnell J, Davis NL. Drug Overdose Deaths Among Persons Aged 10-19 Years – United States, July 2019-December 2021. *MMWR Morb Mortal Wkly Rep* 2022; 71:1576-1582.

Spencer MR, Miniño AM, Warner M. Drug overdose deaths in the United States, 2001–2021. NCHS Data Brief, no 457. Hyattsville, MD: National Center for Health Statistics. 2022. CDC.gov website. Dec-2022. doi. org/10.15620/cdc:122556

Xu JQ, Murphy SL, Kochanek KD, Arias E. Mortality in the United States, 2021. NCHS Data Brief, no 456. Hyattsville, MD: National Center for Health Statistics. 2022. doi.org/10.15620/cdc:122516 (Accessed 23-Dec-2022).

Bruzelius E, Martins SS. US Trends in Drug Overdose Mortality Among Pregnant and Postpartum Persons, 2017-2020. *J Am Med Assoc.* 2022; 328(21):2159-2161.

National Center for Health Statistics. Fentanyl Overdose Death Rates More Than Tripled From 2016 to 2021. CDC.gov website. 3-May-2023. (Accessed 5-Jun-2023).

Jeffery MM, Stevens M, D'Onofrio G, Melnick ER. Fentanyl-Associated Overdose Deaths Outside the Hospital. *N Engl J Med.* 2023; 389:87-88.

CDC Press Release about 2021 Overdose Deaths

Centers for Disease Control and Prevention. Press Release: "U.S. Overdose Deaths In 2021 Increased Half as Much as in 2020 – But Are Still Up 15%." CDC.gov website. 11-May-2022. (Accessed 13-May-2022).

Projection of Future Opioid Deaths

Humphreys K, Shover CL, Andrews CM, Bohnert ASB, Brandeau ML, Caulkins JP, et al. Responding to the opioid crisis in North America and beyond: recommendations of the Stanford–Lancet Commission. *Lancet.* 2022; 399:555-603.

Costs of Opioid Use Disorder and Overdose Deaths

Luo F, Li M, Florence C. State-Level Economic Costs of Opioid Use Disorder and Fatal Opioid Overdose – United States, 2017. *MMWR Morb Mortal Wkly Rep.* 2021; 70(15):541-546.

Cancer Deaths

Siegel RL, Miller KD, Fuchs H, Jemal A. Cancer Statistics, 2021. *CA Cancer J Clin.* 2021; 71:7-33.

Firearm and Automobile Deaths

Centers for Disease Control and Prevention. All Injuries. CDC.gov website. 21-Oct-2021. (Accessed 10-Jan-2022).

Conditions for Providers and Patients Receiving Opioid Treatment

Coffin PO, Barreveld AM. Inherited Patients Taking Opioids for Chronic Pain – Considerations for Primary Care. *N Engl J Med.* 2022; 386:611-613.

Szalavitz M. "What the Opioid Crisis Took From People in Pain." *New York Times.* 7-Mar-2022. (Accessed 10-Mar-2022).

Bipartisan Opioid Commission Report

Commission on Combating Synthetic Opioid Trafficking. Final Report. Rand.org website. 2-Feb-2022. p.2, xv. (Accessed 9-Feb-2022).

Chapter Twelve – Putting an End to Horrific Facts

2022 CDC Updated Opioid Prescription Guideline

Centers for Disease Control and Prevention. Updated Draft CDC Guideline for Prescribing Opioids. Regulations.gov website. 10-Feb-2022. (Accessed 28-Feb-2022).

Dowell D, Ragan KR, Jones CM, Baldwin GT, Chou R. CDC Clinical Practice Guideline for Prescribing Opioids for Pain – United States, 2022. *MMWR Recomm Rep.* 2022; 71(No. RR-3):1-95.

CDC Media Statements about 2022 CDC Updated Opioid Guideline

Centers for Disease Control and Prevention. Press Release: "Federal Register Notice: CDC's updated Clinical Practice Guideline for Prescribing Opioids is now open for public comment – Media Statement." CDC.gov website. 10-Feb-2022. (Accessed 28-Feb-2022).

Centers for Disease Control and Prevention. Press Release: "CDC Releases UPDATED Clinical Practice Guideline for Prescribing Opioids for Pain." CDC.gov website. 3-Nov-2022. (Accessed 12-Nov-2022).

NEJM Perspective Article about 2022 CDC Opioid Guideline

Dowell D, Ragan KR, Jones CM, Baldwin GT, Chou R. Prescribing Opioids for Pain – The New CDC Practice Guideline. *N Engl J Med.* 2022; 387:2011-2013.

Media Reports about 2022 CDC Updated Opioid Guideline

Bernstein L. "CDC proposes new prescription opioid guidelines for caregivers." *Washington Post.* 10-Feb-2022. (Accessed 28-Feb-2022).

Alltucker K. "Amid backlash from chronic pain sufferers, CDC drops hard thresholds from opioid guidance." *USA TODAY.* 10-Feb-2022. (Accessed 28-Feb-2022).

Hoffman J. "C.D.C. Proposes New Guidelines for Treating Pain, Including Opioid Use." *New York Times.* 10-Feb-2022. (Accessed 28-Feb-2022).

Stobbe M. "CDC proposes softer guidance on opioid prescriptions." *AP News.* AP News.com website. 10-Feb-2022. (Accessed 28-Feb-2022).

Anson P. "Revised CDC Opioid Guideline Gives Doctors More Flexibility." *Pain News Network.* Pain News Network.org website. 10-Feb-2022. (Accessed 10-Mar-2022).

Stone W, Huang P. "CDC issues new opioid prescribing guidance, giving doctors more leeway to treat pain." *National Public Radio (NPR).* NPR.org website. 3-Nov-2022. (Accessed 12-Nov-2022).

Brooks M. "New CDC Guidance on Prescribing Opioids for Pain." Medscape.com website. 3-Nov-2022. (Accessed 12-Nov-2022).

Joseph A. "New CDC opioid guidelines emphasize flexibility in treating pain." *STAT.* Statnews.com website. 3-Nov-2022. (Accessed 12-Nov-2022).

Bernstein L. "CDC releases new, more flexible guidelines for prescribing opioids." *Washington Post.* 3-Nov-2022. (Accessed 12-Nov-2022).

Continued Difficulties for Chronic Pain Patients Accessing Pain Treatment

Whitehead S, Miller A. "Chronic pain patients struggle to get opioid prescriptions filled, even as CDC eases guidelines." CNN.com website. 17-Mar-2023. (Accessed 5-Jun-2023).

Darbha V, King L, Westbrook A. "They Live in Constant Pain, but Their Doctors Won't Help Them." *New York Times*. 17-Aug-2023. (Accessed 26-Aug-2023).

Durbhakula S. "The D.E.A. Needs to Stay Out of Medicine." *New York Times*. 22-Mar-2024. (Accessed 22-Mar-2024).

New "Get Tough" Laws for Opioid Possession

Ovalle D. "'War on drugs' deja vu: Fentanyl overdoses spur states to seek tougher laws." *Washington Post*. 6-Apr-2023. (Accessed 5-Jun-2023).

Hoffman J. "Harsh New Fentanyl Laws Ignite Debate Over How To Combat Overdose Crisis." *New York Times*. 21-Jun-2023. (Accessed 25-Jun-2023).

2022 Overdose Estimate

National Center for Health Statistics. Provisional Data Shows U.S. Drug Overdose Deaths Top 100,000 in 2022. CDC.gov website. 18-May-2023. (Accessed 5-Jun-2023).

Weiland N. "U.S. Recorded Nearly 110,000 Overdose Deaths in 2022." *New York Times*. 17-May-2023. (Accessed 5-Jun-2023).

Jeffrey MM, Stevens M, D'Onofrio G, Melnick ER. Fentanyl-Associated Overdose Deaths Outside the Hospital. *N Engl J Med*. 2023; 389:87-88.

DEA on Opioid Public Health Emergency

Diversion Control Division, Drug Enforcement Administration. End of COVID Public Health Emergency (PHE) beginning of Opioid (PHE) May 11, 2023. Email to DEA registrants. 11-May-2023.

2022-2024 CDC Budgets

Centers for Disease Control and Prevention. FY 2024 Congressional Justification. CDC.gov website. 13-Mar-2023. (Accessed 5-Jun-2023).

Chapter Thirteen – Confessions of a Narc Pusher in Appalachia

Tribal Health Care and Narcotic Issues

Ridderbusch K. "How The Eastern Cherokee Took Control Of Their Health Care." *Kaiser Health News*. KFF Health News.org website. 22-Jul-2019. (Accessed 28-Jun-2023).

"Drilling into DEA's pain pill database." *Washington Post*. 21-Jul-2019. Jackson County & Swain County, North Carolina. (Accessed 25-Aug-2019).

McDonald T. "America's Drug Problem Hits Home for North Carolina's Cherokee Tribe." *Raleigh News & Observer*. TheCrimeReport.org website. 13-May-2019. (Accessed 28-Aug-2019).

Hoffman J. "Tribes Reach $590 Million Opioid Settlement With J. & J. and Distributors." *New York Times*. 1-Feb-2022. (Accessed 3-Feb-2022).

Kariisa M, Davis NL, Kumar S, Seth P, Mattson CL Chowdhury F, et al. Vital Signs: Drug Overdose Deaths, by Selected Sociodemographic and Social Determinants of Health Characteristics – 25 States and the District of Columbia, 2019-2020. *MMWR Morb Mortal Wkly Rep*. 2022; 71:940-947.

Tobacco Settlement

"Where did all that tobacco settlement money go?" *Industrial Safety & Hygiene News*. ISHN.com website. 24-Dec-2019. (Accessed 14-Jun-2023).

Campaign for Tobacco-Free Kids. "A State-by-State Look at the 1998 Tobacco Settlement 24 Years Later." Tobacco Free Kids.org website. 13-Jan-2023. (Accessed 14-Jun-2023).

Opioid Settlements

Hoffman J. "Purdue Pharma Is Dissolved and Sacklers Pay $4.5 Billion to Settle Opioid Claims." *New York Times*. 17-Sep-2021. (Accessed 14-Jun-2023).

Hoffman J. "An Appeals Court Gave the Sacklers Legal Immunity. Here's What the Ruling Means." *New York Times*. 31-May-2023. (Accessed 14-Jun-2023).

Hoffman J. "Opioid Settlement Money Is Being Spent on Police Cars and Overtime." *New York Times*. 14-Aug-2023. (Accessed 26-Aug-2023).

Pattani A, Beard M. "Why opioid settlement money is paying county employees' salaries." *Washington Post*. 16-Apr-2024. (Accessed 17-Apr-2024).

Afterword

Number of Persons with Opioid Use Disorder and Proportion Treated

Substance Abuse and Mental Health Services Administration. Key substance use and mental health indicators in the United States: Results from the 2022 National Survey on Drug Use and Health (HHS Publication No. PEP23-07-01-006, NSDUH Series H-58). Center for Behavioral Health Statistics and Quality, Substance Abuse and Mental Health Services Administration Nov-2023. (Accessed 9-Mar-2024).

Need for Opioid Use Disorder Treatment to Control Opioid Epidemic

Commission on Combating Synthetic Opioid Trafficking. Final Report. Rand.org website. 2-Feb-2022. p.xiii. (Accessed 9-Feb-2022).

Effect of Supply-Side-Only Interventions

Szalavitz M. "People Can't Get Their A.D.H.D. Medicine, and That's a Sign of a Larger Problem." *New York Times.* 23-Mar-2023. (Accessed 6-Jun-2023).

Dasgupta N. We Can't Arrest Our Way Out of Overdose: The Drug Bust Paradox. *Am J Public Health.* 2023; 113:708.

Opioid Use Disorder Treatment Compared with Treatment for Other Chronic Conditions

McLellan AT, Lewis DC, O'Brien CP, Kleber HD. Drug Dependence, a Chronic Medical Illness: Implications for Treatment, Insurance, and Outcomes Evaluation. *J Am Med Assoc.* 2000; 284(13):1689-1695.

Annual Mortality from Alcohol Use

Esser MB, Sherk A, Liu Y, Naimi TS. Deaths from Excessive Alcohol Use — United States, 2016—2021. *MMWR Morb Mortal Wkly Rep* 2024; 73:154-161.

Annual and Lifetime Mortality from Smoking

Centers for Disease Control and Prevention. Smoking and Tobacco Use: Fast Facts. CDC.gov website. 4-May-2023. (Accessed 28-Jun-2023).

Banks E, Joshy G, Weber MF, Liu B, Grenfell R, Egger S, et al. Tobacco smoking and all-cause mortality in a large Australian cohort study: findings from a mature epidemic with current low smoking prevalence. *BMC Med.* 2015; 13:38. doi.org/10.1186/s12916-015-0281-z

Cost-Effectiveness of Opioid Use Disorder Treatment

Fairley M, Humphreys K, Joyce VR, Bounthavong M, Trafton J, Combs A, et al. Cost-effectiveness of Treatments for Opioid Use Disorder. *JAMA Psychiatry.* 2021; 78(7):767-777.

Proportion of U.S. Adults With Family Who Died of Overdoses

Sparks G, Montero A, Kirzinger A. "KFF Tracking Poll July 2023: Substance Use Crisis and Access Treatment." KFF.org website. 15-Aug-2023. (Accessed 26-Aug-2023).

Epigraphs

Boethius. *The Consolation of Philosophy.* Translated by David R. Slavitt Cambridge, MA. Harvard University Press. 2008. Book 1, Section VI.

Mary Tyler Moore. Variation on "You can't be brave if you've only had wonderful things happen to you." Brucculieri J. "Mary Tyler Moore Quotes To Remember During Challenging Times." *Huff Post.* 25-Jan-2017. (Accessed 1-Sep-2021).

William Foege. In: Baggett L. "No one will thank you for the disease they didn't get." *UGA News.* News.uga.edu website. 3-Oct-2018. (Accessed 1-Sep-2021).

Jean de La Bruyère, *Les Caractères.* Malesherbes, France: Folio Classique. 2016. "Du Coeur #77." p.93.

Rickey Henderson. Wikipedia.org website. (Accessed 20-Jul-2022).

George Wald. "Science Quotes by George Wald." Today in Science History (TodayInSci.com) website. [No date]. (Accessed 1-Sep-2021).

Joseph Roth. *The Radetzky March.* Translated by Joachim Neugroschel. New York, NY: The Overlook Press, Abrams Books; 2021. p.111.

John Gay. *The Beggar's Opera.* The Beggar's Opera and Other Eighteenth Century Plays. Rutland, VT: Everyman Library, J.M.Dent; 1995. p.167.

ABOUT THE AUTHOR

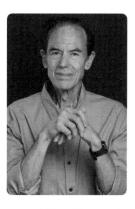

Bonnie J. Heath Photography

For more than twenty-eight years, Charles LeBaron worked as a medical epidemiologist at the Centers for Disease Control and Prevention (CDC), where he was the author of more than fifty scientific studies published in peer-reviewed journals, including first- or senior-author papers published in the *New England Journal of Medicine* and the *Journal of the American Medical Association.* He was co-recipient of CDC's Charles C. Shepard Science Award for best scientific manuscript published by CDC authors. A Captain in the Commissioned Corps of the United States Public Health Service, he received the Meritorious Service Medal, as well as more than ten other individual and unit commendation awards. A graduate of Princeton University and Harvard Medical School, he is board certified in both internal medicine and pediatrics, as well as the author of a previous non-fiction account of the first year of medical school. He currently lives in Atlanta, Georgia.

FOR THE HEROES
WITH NO NAMES

The unacknowledged heroes of the opioid epidemic are too many to salute here, from solitary rehab workers in rural treatment deserts to EMTs in urban addiction zones. It would be wrong, however, if this book ended without recognition of two equivalently anonymous groups:

–The line staff at CDC's Division of Overdose Prevention who, despite the issues chronicled in the pages above, work to make a positive impact on the nation's overdose crisis, trying their best to provide high-quality data to guide life-saving public health policy, an objective which a long-ago CDC Director identified as the agency's first, true, and overriding priority. And still should be. Those line workers carry the torch.

–The courageous, grieving families who give an unforgettable human face to the epidemic by sharing with the world the photographic portraits of loved ones who were stolen from them by overdoses and whose joys and worries and dreams in life are so achingly visible. Without the families' bravery, all the statistical columns and rows might mean nothing to us but inert numbers. Those families make us understand why we must learn from the numbers and find the strength to act.

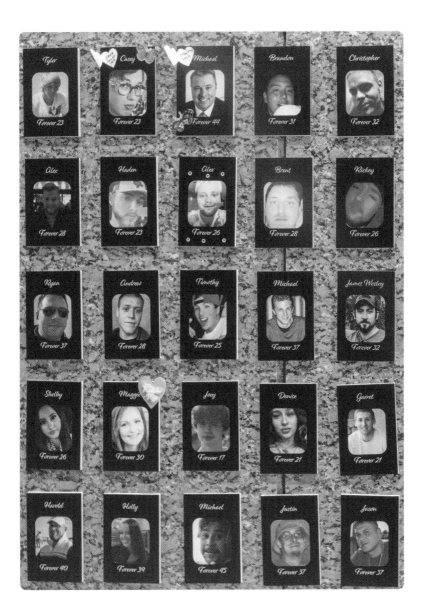

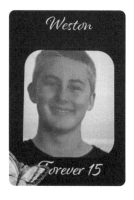
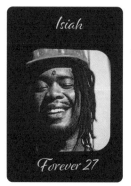
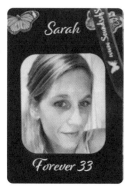
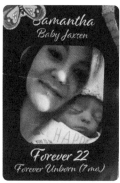
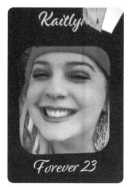
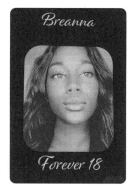

Portraits of a few of the million victims of fatal overdoses remembered
by families in the U.S. Drug Enforcement Administration (DEA) public
exhibit "Faces of Fentanyl." (www.dea.gov/fentanylawareness)
Photographs of the exhibit by John Canan

BEN. So, it seems, his time was come.
JEMMY. But the present time is ours, and
nobody alive hath more.

   – John Gay (1685-1732), *The Beggar's Opera*

.